HOW TO KEEP
MOM
(AND YOURSELF)
OUT OF
A NURSING HOME

Seven Keys to Keeping
Your Independence

D1445741

DAVID FISHER, MD

For Jean, my inspiration
My home is forever with you

How to Keep Mom (and Yourself) Out of a Nursing Home:
Seven Keys to Keeping Your Independence

ISBN-10: 0-984420-20-7
ISBN-13: 978-0-984420-20-9

Printed in the United States of America

CONTENTS

ACKNOWLEDGEMENTS

I thank God for the vision, inspiration, and resources that animated this project. May the work of my hands, infused by your strength, bless many people for your glory.

To my bride, Jean, every day you encourage me to believe in the gifts God gives. You are his greatest gift to me. Your selfless sacrifices made this project possible. You are the seal that holds our family together. Thank you for knowing how to inspire me. Very few men have experienced the type of soul nurture that I enjoy in your presence. It is a blessing to walk this life with you.

To my children, thank you for your endless encouragement and patience with the project known as "Dad's book." Hannah, one smile from you is enough to brighten the darkest day. Your beauty is rooted in your unwavering hope. Isaac, your steady confidence points me toward faith in the seemingly impossible. Your fearlessness inspires me. Ian, you invigorate me with your boundless energy. Your vitality is contagious.

To my mother-in-law, thank you for your steady presence in the midst of intermittent chaos. Your prayers and grace, rooted in your deep faith, are a strong anchor and I am forever grateful.

To my parents, thank you for your prayers, your support, and for encouraging my joy of writing.

To the Szalays, the family corn farm is the first place where I observed successful and graceful aging, in my grandparents and in the entire family. Thank you for setting an example of healthy living through joyful, intergenerational, and purposeful activity.

To Dewey and Alison Snowden, thank you for your words of encouragement.

To Kathy Wone, thank you for your thoughtful feedback. To Frank Gutbrod, your patience and creativity made the vision a reality.

To Steve Raquel and Chanda Dies, thank you for accompanying me into the increasingly complicated world of multimedia.

To Paul, Peter, Bethany, and your families, thank you for your prayers and for your cheerleading.

To Richard Segal, thank you for continually reminding me of the truth.

To our faithful friends at Redeemer, Covenant and Calvary churches, your prayers cleared the way through many a dark tunnel and unexpected bend in the road.

To the Cru Zoo, thanks for the laughter and friendship.

Finally, to my physician mentors, I am deeply grateful. Janice Benson showed a young medical student how to listen. Richard Lord taught the art of talking with patients, not at them. Jeff Williamson, Hal Atkinson, Kaycee Sink, Mary Lyles and Chip Celestino refined my practice of geriatric medicine. Richard Stephenson exhibited the kindness and honesty that turns a doctor-patient conversation from a mere exchange of information into a "heart to heart."

CHAPTER ONE

YOU NEED A PLAN

The first thing you need to know about nursing homes is this: *you don't want to live in one.* As a nursing home physician, I have observed the slow and tragic decline these institutions inflict on their residents. This is not intentional; most nursing facilities spend millions of dollars and incorporate the efforts of dozens of thoughtful individuals in an attempt to serve their residents well. Nevertheless, institutional living by its very nature often leads to a downward spiral in almost every facet of health, whether physical, mental, emotional or spiritual. Furthermore, numerous unintended forces exist in nursing homes that can severely restrict a resident's chance of ever leaving. The primary purpose of this book is to help you or your loved one avoid the nursing home trap.

Why Nursing Homes Exist

In the popular movie *The Bucket List*, starring Jack Nicholson and Morgan Freeman, two aging men make a list of things they would like to do before they die, or "kick the bucket." They visit exotic places, go skydiving, and make amends with estranged loved ones. Not surprisingly, "to live in a nursing home" is nowhere on their list. Indeed, no one I know plans or hopes to end up in a nursing home. Most children of aging parents claim that no matter what, they will do whatever is necessary to keep mom or dad "out of a home." Yet, in 2008, the US Census reports that almost 1.7 million Americans live in a nursing home. If none of the residents planned to, then why do so many people end up there? The answer can be summarized in three words: *loss of independence*. Loss of independence is the primary reason that you or a loved one will need future care in a nursing home.

Personal independence and self-determination are two of our most coveted values. Thomas Jefferson ranked the right to liberty (i.e. personal independence) and the pursuit of happiness (i.e. self-determination) on the same level with life itself. Health and independence are deeply intertwined; we pursue better health as a means to increase our chances of controlling our own destinies. For example, why do people monitor their blood pressure and cholesterol? There is no immediate payoff to lowering the systolic pressure by a few points or knocking out a few of the low density lipoproteins (LDLs) circulating through our bloodstream; we feel the same whether our cholesterol is 160 or 245. Yet, we acknowledge that doing what we can now to avoid a heart attack or stroke later will keep us out of the hospital, off of medications, and will allow us to go and do what we want when we want. Do we sometimes run or swim the extra lap for the pure joy of it? Yes, but more often than not, the extra effort now is simply to let us justify some extra dessert later on. In the same way, we pursue better health now so we can remain independent later.

So what does independence have to do with living in a nursing home? Everything. Every person who lives in a nursing home needs help with some daily activity, but they did not have the resources to get that help at home. The activities they need help with are those we often take for granted: eating, bathing, grooming, walking or getting out of bed, and toileting. These daily necessities to independent living have been defined as the Activities of Daily Living, or "ADL's". Much of this book will explore strategies for maintaining ADL function as the primary means to stay out of a nursing home. People who cannot independently perform their ADLs will quickly end up in a nursing home.

Aging is Not the Enemy

I am a medical doctor who specializes in geriatrics, the specialty that focuses on aging. Thanks to tremendous medical advances over the past century, people are living longer than ever. The quest for youth continues to invade our nation's consciousness. We cannot turn on the TV or open a magazine without hearing about the latest anti-aging diet or lifestyle. Incredible and promising research is being done that will continue to extend the average human lifespan, and some experts are predicting advances in longevity that we never would have thought possible even twenty years ago. While this progress is exciting, a longer life by itself is not the ultimate goal.

If I told you that you could live to be one hundred and fifty, would you be overjoyed or would you worry? When I ask my patients if they want me to help them live longer, they will inevitably answer yes, but they will always add some type of qualifier, such as:

"Sure, doc, as long as I still have my wits about me."

"Absolutely, provided I'm not in a lot of pain."

"Definitely, as long as I can still go bowling."

"Yes, but if I ever have to move to a nursing home, I'm not so sure."A longer life is not the real goal here. *Length* of life is only worthwhile if it is coupled with *quality of life.*

What gives us quality of life? The contributing factors are many, whether it is doing things we enjoy, spending meaningful time with family and friends, the feeling that we are contributing to society, or the ability to foster and maintain our spiritual growth. When we talk about "staying young" or maintaining our "quality of life", what we are really talking about is independence, keeping some level of control and autonomy over our own lives. To lose our independence is to lose our very humanity.

The science of geriatrics defines healthy aging by one's ability to function independently. Aging tends to rob us of our independence. Losing the ability to drive, for example, can be a brutal blow to the previously independent adult. Aging causes a steady decline in our independent function, beginning with more advanced skills such as driving a car or operating a business and culminating in the loss of the most basic human functions such as the ability to independently use the bathroom or feed ourselves. Those who have cared for an aging loved one can testify to the devastating toll taken by this long, painful process.

In my practice, I have admitted thousands of people to nursing homes. I have heard the same stories over and over as patients and their families describe the specific factors and events that led to loss of independence and subsequent placement in a nursing home. From those stories emerge a few well-defined pathways that will inevitably lead to nursing home placement. Insight into these pathways cannot be gleaned from poring over facility admission records or reviewing Medicare data. Understanding why people end up in nursing homes is best achieved by listening to their stories, something I do everyday as a physician. I hope to share that knowledge with you so that you and your loved ones can avoid the common pitfalls into which many of my patients have unwittingly fallen.

The Keys to Independence

As we battle the toll that aging takes on the body, spirit, and larger community, we need to redefine the enemy. As mentioned earlier, the enemy is not aging. It is the loss of independence. How do we fight from losing our independence? Is the answer found in a diet, a vitamin, a martial art, or a medical procedure? Prominent physicians have devoted entire careers to slowing the aging process, and I hope this research continues. Unfortunately, many of us are already dealing with the impact of a chronic disease on our health or the health of a loved one. Despite our best efforts to adhere to the recommended healthy habits, we are all likely to develop one or more age-related chronic conditions or illnesses. Further, maintaining health takes time and resources. It is difficult to sift through the enormous amount of information available today and determine what health recommendations are most important to follow.

This book will give you a strategic plan that focuses on maintaining the aspects of health that are most important to independent living. The field of geriatrics research ranges widely, from exploring the genetic causes of aging to understanding the characteristics of people who live one hundred or more years. I have relied heavily on the aspects of geriatric research that emphasize the practical nature of daily function. For example, to stay out of a nursing home, is it more important to have strong biceps or a strong external urinary sphincter muscle? The answer may surprise you.

For those who are the picture of health, you will learn where to continue focusing your efforts. For those who are beginning to feel the effects of aging, you will learn to identify warning signs and how to respond in a way that maximizes your efforts toward maintaining independence. And for those who are on the brink of needing nursing home care, you will read about the pitfalls that could ultimately place you in one and what specific steps you can still take to avoid leaving your precious home.

As a physician specializing in geriatrics, I want to put myself out of a job. While I enjoy interacting with my patients who live in various nursing homes, I am distressed by the number of people who probably could have avoided ever being admitted. I have met many wonderful people who needed this book just a few years, or even a few months, earlier. Unfortunately, age-related health crises will be impossible to eliminate and there will always be a need for nursing home care. I pray that with the help of this book, you will be able to choose a better story for yourself or your loved one.

CHAPTER TWO

IT'S NOT THE AGING,
IT'S THE
INDEPENDENCE

Consider the ways of the ant, and be wise. Without having
any chief officer, or ruler, she prepares her bread in summer and
gathers her food in harvest.

- Hebrew proverb

Most Americans prepare for retirement. Money is usually the first thing that comes to mind when we think of retirement planning. We shop for the best mutual funds, strategize about our 401(k), and give full-time jobs to financial planners who help us pile up the right amount of financial resources by a certain age. We presume that these resources will give us control over the remaining years of our lives. Unfortunately, retirement planning is often based on the assumption that independence can be guaranteed with money.

Think of all the planning and effort that goes into preparing our bank accounts for retirement. Now imagine if we put the same amount of effort into preparing our bodies for retirement.

We work long, hard hours while we are younger and healthier because we know that a time will come when we may not be able to work. We also look forward to a time when we will no longer have to work. We try to save enough so that our financial ledger has the necessary reserve to handle life without needing a steady income. In the same way, your body carries a certain level of *reserve* at any one moment. The key to preparing your body for retirement is amassing the right amount of *reserve*.

A Retirement Plan for Your Body: Reserve is the Key

Did you know that your body can function with one kidney? Or that your liver can adequately do its job at 25% capacity? The average adult has a large amount of built-in reserve. Most of our organ systems give us more than we need for everyday survival. Our bodies may call upon this reserve during a particularly stressful event, such as a sudden trauma or serious infection. Only in such extreme situations does it become evident how much capacity our bodies are actually carrying.

As we age, our reserve begins to disappear. Unfortunately, we often lose a lot of our reserve without even knowing it. As long as we only ask the minimum of our bodies, we can function on very little of our true capacity. Meanwhile, the added reserve contained within an organ system can decline without warning. If we don't know what to look for, it will take a crisis to uncover a critical drop in reserve.

Let's examine the kidneys as an example. Bill and Joe appear equally healthy on the outside. Bill's kidneys are functioning at 100%, while Joe's are only functioning at 40%

due to years of high blood pressure. Unless Joe's doctor orders blood tests to measure his kidney function, it is unlikely that Joe would be aware of his reduced kidney capacity. His kidneys can still function adequately for day-to-day living, even at 40%. However, subject Joe and Bill to a urinary tract infection and a couple of days of low fluid intake, and Joe could become dehydrated and teeter on the brink of kidney failure. Meanwhile Bill's kidneys may temporarily drop to 85 or 90 percent capacity, but he wouldn't even know the difference.

Stop Living Paycheck to Paycheck

Asking our bodies for only the minimum is like living paycheck to paycheck. It is possible to survive for months or even years this way, but when the reserve is tapped out, just one unexpected event can turn into a major catastrophe. Like our bank accounts, our bodies should be prepared not only for the next 2 weeks, but for the unforeseen future. In planning for your body's retirement, it is important to think of your body as your physical bank account, but with two key differences.

The first difference is the rate of investment. Most people start their first savings account with a small amount of money. I started mine as a teenager with birthday gift money I had collected over the years, which only amounted to a few hundred dollars. Over the years, however, I have been able to increase the amount I save per month, allowing me to build that wealth gradually. I will need to continue this pattern of saving until I retire if I want to reach my goal.

It is different with our bodies. When we reach adulthood, we are blessed with a large initial investment in our reserve that we did nothing to achieve. The growing process gives us strong muscles, bones, and brains that will last us for years without any special effort on our part. It is the financial equivalent of receiving a large trust fund upon graduating from college. With proper management, that large reserve can last a lifetime. Instead of scraping and scrimping for years in order to save the body's reserve, all that is required is good maintenance. We don't need to get our bodies into marathon-running shape to prepare for the future, but we do need to take care of the reserve we are given because unlike a really good stock pick, our bodies operate on a negative interest rate.

Most retirement accounts boast a good rate of return. The best accounts can offer twelve to fifteen percent per year or higher. With enough reserve, the interest earned on the account is enough to meet our needs week to week; we no longer have to keep putting money into the account in order for it to sustain us.

Not so with our bodies. We have in our bodies a negative interest rate, and this is the second difference between your body's retirement plan and your bank account. The reserve that we were given in our late teens and early twenties begins to disappear over time. As we age, we begin losing that reserve at a much faster rate; what took very little to maintain in our thirties takes much more to maintain in our sixties.. If you had an investment portfolio that was losing money at increasingly faster rates each year, you would become very concerned and sell that fund or change banks. However, we all are stuck with the bodies we were given. We cannot trade or sell our bodies for a better one. Our bodies will continue losing capacity as they age, so the only thing to do is invest in our reserves for as long as we can.

Supplies are Limited, So Act Now

Certain aspects of our reserve can only be stored up while we are young. Just as our income-earning potential is limited by time, the physical factors that support our independence are slowly deteriorating and must be built up while still possible. Similar to a financial retirement plan, planning for *functional independence* requires a strategic investment portfolio that anticipates needs and wants, protects against pitfalls, and diversifies against catastrophe. And just like saving for retirement, the sooner we start on our body's retirement plan, the better.

Financial retirement planning requires us to learn a new language. We learn terms like rollover, tax deferment, annuity, and diversification. We study the concepts of compound interest, employer matching, and estate planning. Those who understand these ideas and the role they play in the larger retirement plan have the best chance of success. Preparing a plan for maintaining your body's independence also requires a new glossary of terms. Mastering a few important concepts will maximize your chances to maintain control over your circumstances as your body ages.

The likelihood that someone will end up in a nursing home depends almost exclusively on how well they can perform a set of daily tasks without help. In the language of geriatric medicine, these tasks are known as the *Activities of Daily*

Living, or ADL, which are the basics of self-care and the focus of this chapter. We cannot maintain functional independence without the ability to perform these essential tasks. Another set of tasks, the *Instrumental Activities of Daily Living* (IADL), further enable us to navigate life within a community. These more advanced tasks are not crucial to staying out of a nursing home, but losing the ability to perform them should be taken as a sign that independence is being threatened. The most successful body retirement plans will focus on these sets of specific tasks and will develop strategies to maintain them for as long as possible.

The Five ADLs

Healthy people usually take for granted their ability get out of bed in the morning, use the bathroom, perform some level of personal hygiene, dress themselves, and feed themselves. These five ADLs are generally considered to be the minimum requirements for daily independence. Once a person starts to lose the ability to perform any one of them, his or her likelihood of moving to a nursing home will skyrocket; therefore, it is crucial that these five skills be maintained.

Toileting and Continence

Our ability to get to and from the bathroom, and the ability to relieve ourselves once in the bathroom, are extremely important to maintaining independence. Losing that ability means losing a large portion of our dignity. Very few people in the early stages of incontinence will volunteer the details about their struggle to family members, close friends, or even to their doctor. Too often, the problem does not come to light until it has reached an unmanageable stage. This is tragic because incontinence is a key factor in requiring nursing home care and preventive steps could have been taken to address the problem in its early stages. The chapter on incontinence will explore this issue in further detail.

Bathing

Bathing is a complicated routine that requires a number of coordinated steps. Proper bathing involves good balance, the ability to reach and bend, and the ability to navigate and control slippery substances and devices. Safety is a key issue in bathing, and many people lose the ability to bathe themselves simply because the risk of injury is too high if they attempt to bathe alone.

Dressing

A key component to dignity in our society is proper dress. An activity that may take a healthy person five minutes can take an hour for someone with diminished motor skills from stroke or arthritis, or diminished cognitive skills due to dementia. If you are unable to dress, it becomes impossible to properly clothe yourself, and it becomes impossible to maintain an independent lifestyle.

Feeding

Acquiring food is not a problem for most people in an industrialized country. Even those who cannot shop or cook for themselves can make arrangements to have meals delivered to their home. However, getting that food from the refrigerator to your mouth is an altogether different matter. If you have lost the ability to feed yourself, your likelihood of needing nursing home placement rises exponentially. One of the most common causes of feeding problems is dementia, and this will be explored in more detail in the chapter on brain function.

Transfer: Getting In and Out of a Bed or Chair

The ability to get up from a seated or lying position is a key to maintaining independence. You can lose the ability to walk and still maintain autonomy; many people with paralysis of the legs lead independent lives, but their independence hinges on their ability to transfer themselves from a bed to a wheelchair and back. Losing the ability to transfer yourself can be a devastating blow to your independence. The causes of this loss are explored further in the chapter on mobility.

Instrumental Activities of Daily Living

The Instrumental Activities of Daily Living, or IADL, are daily tasks that require a higher level of functioning and mark the ability to truly live independently. They include the ability to use the telephone, to shop, prepare food, maintain the house, do laundry, arrange for one's own transportation, manage one's medications, and handle one's finances.

Loss of IADL function can be addressed mostly through social support systems, such as family, religious, or municipal resources. Losing the ability to perform these tasks does not necessarily mean that nursing home care will be required. Many people who maintain ADL function but have difficulty with certain IADLs have arranged to live in a senior living facility or assisted living facility. Details about the different types of long term care facilities can be found in Chapter 8.

Your Investment Strategy

Get started today on your retirement plan for your body. Now that you understand the key functional components of independence, this book will further help you identify areas of attention that will maximize your time and efforts as you prepare for the future. Whether you are healthy or already shopping around for nursing homes, you need a plan that has the best chance of success. Let me help you make some strategic investments that will really pay off.

ACTION STEPS

▣ Take the Independence Assessment Questionnaires (appendix A)

CHAPTER THREE

PEOPLE IN MOTION
STAY IN MOTION

Evelyn, age seventy-two, lived in a two-story home with John, her husband of 48 years. They had three children. Evelyn developed diabetes in her forties, and she managed the disease for 35 years with moderate success. Over the past two years, she had been suffering from burning pain in her feet caused by diabetic neuropathy. In addition, her bladder control was falling victim to overflow incontinence, a common consequence of diabetes that results in embarrassing leaking episodes that can occur without warning.

Evelyn was overweight, and her knees bore the majority of the burden for decades. Now she felt the constant pain of osteoarthritis as the bones in her knee joints ground together. Simple, daily activities like descending the stairs or getting in and out of a chair became difficult chores. John, age seventy-five, had some heart problems, and it became too much for him to help Evelyn around the house every day.

Their oldest daughter, Grace, and her husband, Dave, were going through some financial difficulties at the time, so the family decided that Grace and Dave would sell their house and move in with John and Evelyn to help out. The plan seemed to work well for a while. They each were able to help Evelyn stand up to her rolling walker when she needed to move about, and Evelyn could now have her meals and other items brought to her. Evelyn liked the new arrangement, but she was doing less and less with her legs, causing her muscles to lose strength.

One day, her husband helped Evelyn outside to walk in their small garden. John turned around and before he knew it, Evelyn was on the ground. It happened so fast. Grace rushed out to help John get Evelyn back on her feet. Luckily, she only sustained a few bruises and was not seriously hurt. The episode unnerved the whole family. Taking walks outside seemed too risky from then on. Evelyn's balance was much worse, resulting from the neuropathy in her feet, and her arthritic knees were no longer able to bear her frame. Evelyn now spent most of her time either in her favorite chair or in bed.

Evelyn was taking medications for heart failure and her occasional chest pains, but one night she became so short of breath that John called 911. The emergency room doctor diagnosed Evelyn with an exacerbation of congestive heart failure, and she was admitted to the hospital. After a few days of intravenous medication, her breathing felt much better, but lying in a hospital bed for just a few days cost her leg muscles much of their remaining strength. Evelyn transferred to a rehabilitation facility to undergo physical therapy. Unfortunately, her arthritis pain prevented her from being able to participate in the type of intensive strengthening program covered by her Medicare insurance, so she was transferred to a nursing home for long-term care. The nurses were so busy that they hardly had time to help Evelyn to the bathroom, not to mention help her exercise her legs every day. Evelyn began to wonder if the small room with the uncomfortable bed was destined to be her new home.

Keep Moving

The scenario described above illustrates Isaac Newton's first law of thermodynamics: an object in motion stays in motion, and an object at rest stays at rest. This law of inertia sheds light on why people end up needing nursing home care. Anyone who spends time in a nursing home will notice that many of the residents living there have a hard time moving around. They may lack the strength to get out of bed themselves or have partial paralysis from a stroke. They may have balance problems from neuropathy caused by diabetes or Parkinson's disease. Whatever the cause, when a person stops moving like they used to, the odds of needing nursing home care increase dramatically

Our muscles are designed to move. When we use our muscles, the tiny fibers contract and release, sliding back and forth across each other to shorten or lengthen the muscle in a coordinated fashion. This process causes tiny tears to occur in some of the muscle fibers. The amazing consequence of these micro-injuries or micro-tears to the muscle tissue is that when the fibers grow back, they grow back a little bigger. Lifting weights is nothing more than causing injury to your muscles so that they grow back slightly larger. Anyone who has experienced soreness following an exercise session has felt this muscle damage.

This process is necessary to maintain muscle health. When muscles do not move, they do not remain the same size. They begin to shrink, a process known as muscle atrophy. For example, when you have to wear an arm cast for an extended period of time because of a broken bone, you will notice that when the cast is removed, the arm will be significantly smaller. For a young person, muscle atrophy tends to occur over several weeks. For someone older who has less reserve, however, muscle atrophy begins almost immediately during a period of immobilization. A tremendous amount of strength is lost during even a short hospitalization when the patient must lie in bed for two or three days. As we grow older, regaining this strength will take much longer. This chapter will explore the consequences of mobility loss, the most common causes of lost mobility, and methods to prevent it.

Consequences of Mobility Loss

Loss of mobility can be devastating. The accomplishment of simple tasks required for daily living become seemingly insurmountable. Mobility loss is clearly a significant contributor for needing nursing home care. When we lose the ability to move, we inch that much closer to nursing home placement as we become more likely to fall, become socially isolated, develop functional incontinence, lose our access to medical care, and become unable to maintain our homes.

Falls

Falls are a common predictor of nursing home placement. As mobility declines, we still tend to think that we can do more than we actually can. We do not want to believe that the stairs we used to leap in a few easy bounds now seem unscalable. We have a hard time accepting that we might have to ask someone to sweep the walk for us, a walkway that we have swept countless times. In an admirable attempt to maintain independence, we try to perform these tasks ourselves. Unfortunately, once our usual mobility begins to decline, we tend to overestimate our abilities and put ourselves in risky situations. As I examine a patient in the emergency room who has fallen, I cannot count the number of times I have heard these words: "I guess I just tried to do too much, doc."

Social Isolation

Loss of mobility also contributes to social isolation. Someone who has trouble getting around in and around their own house certainly is no longer prepared to host a group of guests in his home. Getting to and from the car or to public transportation also becomes very difficult. This often leads to depression, and a consequence of depression is a loss of motivation to try and engage in activities one enjoys doing. A vicious cycle develops where the person who was once active is now depressed about his lack of activity ... which leads to further muscle weakening and mobility loss ... which leads to increased depression and decreased motivation ...

Functional Incontinence

A major problem with mobility loss is losing the ability to get to and from the bathroom. You may have perfect bladder and bowel control, but weakness and slow movement makes it extremely difficult to make it to the bathroom in time. This is known as functional incontinence and is explored in more detail in the chapter on incontinence.

Loss of Access to Medical Care

Most people who are losing their mobility also have multiple medical problems. These medical concerns must be closely watched by a physician as an exacerbation of any one of these problems can quickly spiral into a catastrophic event. Unfortunately, lack of mobility often prevents people from getting to and from their doctor's appointments, appointments that could have prevented further illness, injury, or even hospitalization. For example, a person with mobility issues and congestive heart failure who is due for a regular appointment may be "feeling alright" and therefore decides not go through the major hassle of seeing his doctor. Had he kept his appointment, the doctor may have noticed the three pound weight gain, a telltale sign that the patient is retaining fluid and may be due for an exacerbation of the heart failure. Preventive measures could have been taken but instead, one week later the person ends up in the emergency room acutely short of breath and is admitted to the hospital. The cycle begins.

Unfit Living Environment

The ability to maintain your house is very important if you want to continue living at home. Mobility is vital to being able to clean your home, throw away the trash, and maintain the yard. I have met many people who were not able to perform these tasks for several weeks and who unfortunately did not have the resources to hire someone to help them. When someone falls or experiences some other medical event that requires a phone call to 911, the emergency medical technicians often arrive to a house that is in such disarray, it must be deemed by law as "unfit" for living. The person is taken to the hospital and is literally barred from his home until significant changes are made. If that person does not have family or resources that can assist with this, he has no choice but to remain in the nursing home while the municipal authorities condemn his home.

Causes of Mobility Loss

Loss of general mobility can occur for many reasons. Sometimes it occurs suddenly as the result of a traumatic event. Other times it occurs slowly over several years. Identifying the main causes of mobility loss is an important step to preventing its occurrence. The main causes include lack of exercise, stroke, other neurologic causes, pain, hospitalizations, depression, and safety concerns.

Lack of Exercise

As described above, our muscles require movement to maintain function. Like our bones, our muscles will grow and adapt according to what we demand from them. The forearms of a championship arm wrestler are the size of tree trunks because the muscles have responded to the stresses he has placed on them. A regular exercise program is key to maintaining your mobility.

The Institute of Medicine released a report in 2002 recommending one hour of strenuous exercise every day.

When our society was such that most people had to perform hard labor to grow food or make a living, this expectation was easy to fulfill. However, the blessings of a mechanized modern society have brought with them a curse: most of us have a hard time finding the time and motivation to exercise. Placing stress on your body to survive is one thing; it is far more difficult to voluntarily work up a sweat when the basics for life can be obtained without much physical effort.

The average person in the U.S. exercises about 100 minutes per week Not only is this far too little to maintain proper cardiovascular health, a mere 100 minutes per week will not preserve the strength that our muscles will require to support our bodies as we age. Placing stress on our muscles through exercise is essential for survival if we are to maintain the independent quality of life that we currently enjoy. As we age, more obstacles will arise to keep us from moving. Preparing our bodies' reserve for handling these obstacles is a key to maintaining independence.

Stroke

About 700,000 Americans will experience a stroke each year. The chapter on brain function provides details on what a stroke is, why it happens, and methods for preventing stroke. The impact of a stroke falls along a continuum. A minor stroke may cause a temporary loss of speech, memory, or limb function that improves within days to weeks; a major stroke can cause permanent paralysis of an entire side of the body, total loss of the ability to speak or process language, an inability to swallow, or coma. This chapter will focus on how a stroke can impact mobility.

Many strokes cause either partial or total loss of motor function on one side of the body. Sometimes the stroke will cause complete paralysis of an arm, leg, or both. Other times, the stroke will cause significant weakness that improves over time. Unfortunately, weakness that is brought on by a stroke often robs the victim of independent mobility. The impact of a stroke, and strategies for preventing strokes, are discussed further in the chapter on vascular health.

Pain

Muscles may be strong enough and balance may be adequate, but joints that are painful to move cause a major problem with mobility. Arthritic joints are perhaps the most common cause of pain that limits mobility. The two most common types of arthritis that limit mobility are osteoarthritis and rheumatoid arthritis. Both forms of joint inflammation are hereditary, but they can also be exacerbated by other factors.

Osteoarthritis occurs when cartilage, the protective cushion that rests between the bones at a joint, begins to wear down. This cartilage cushion is like a tire tread that wears away over time. When it becomes thin enough, the bones begin to rub together, causing painful inflammation in the joint. Once osteoarthritis sets in, it becomes difficult to cure. The most common sites of osteoarthritis are the knees and hip joints. It may also occur in the wrists, hands, and spine, especially in the neck, where the cartilage padding between the vertebral bones is smaller.

Most doctors will prescribe anti-inflammatory medications for osteoarthritis in its early stages. This medicine reduces the inflammation in the joint and makes the pain more manageable.

It does nothing, however, to improve the underlying condition. Many doctors recommend that people with heart disease, high blood pressure, acid reflux, or stomach ulcers not take anti-inflammatory medications on a long-term basis. A reasonable alternative is acetaminophen (the generic for Tylenol) three or four times a day. Again, this treatment provides a level of pain control that allows patients to maintain mobility, but it does not solve the underlying problem.

Steroid injections or synthetic joint fluid can provide significant relief to an arthritic joint. Unfortunately, this relief usually lasts for a few months at best, and these procedures can only be performed two or three times altogether. People with severe cases of osteoarthritis may undergo joint replacement surgery, usually performed on the knee or the hip. Patients with complicated medical problems such as heart disease will not qualify for this type of surgery, and candidates for joint replacement must have a realistic chance to successfully undergo a period of rehabilitation that may last anywhere from four to eight weeks or longer.

Rheumatoid arthritis is an autoimmune disorder that affects the joints, usually in the hands and fingers. An autoimmune disease is a condition that occurs when the body's natural immune system becomes confused. A healthy immune system is designed to attack foreign objects that enter our body. When a virus or bacteria invades our system, the antibodies and immune cells that make up this defense system will rush to the invaders and destroy them. This process naturally causes inflammation, resulting in heat, swelling, and pain. When the immune system is fighting an enemy, these are necessary side effects of the inflammatory response.

Autoimmune disorders occur when the immune system confuses normal, healthy tissue for a foreign substance and attacks it. In rheumatoid arthritis, tissues in the joint are attacked by the confused immune system, causing inflammation. This debilitating disease can be treated with certain anti-inflammatories like steroids, but many people continue to suffer from this disease despite the most current treatments. Rheumatoid arthritis that affects the hands can severely limit someone's ability to perform their ADLs independently. It is less common for rheumatoid arthritis to affect the legs or feet but when it does, mobility becomes severely limited.

Hospitalization

Lying in a hospital bed will cause a significant loss of muscle strength. Even a seventy-two hour stay in a hospital can result in profound weakness. Unfortunately, hospitalized patients have many obstacles to getting up and moving around. For example, they are often hooked up to intravenous lines or monitoring machines that make it difficult to get out of bed. Frequent staff visits to check vital signs or draw blood make sleeping difficult, resulting in daytime exhaustion that leaves one even less energized to move about during the day. For this reason, many who are hospitalized for even a short time will require a short-term stay in a nursing home in order to regain their strength through physical therapy. For those who lack the reserve to participate in physical therapy, all too often the hospitalization is the tipping point from which they will never fully recover. These people often end up staying long term in the nursing home.

Safety Concerns

Those who suffer from lack of strength or lack of balance are, understandably, afraid of falling. Homes that are not equipped to accommodate someone with mobility problems can quickly become safety hazards. There may be floors in the home that have not been visited in months because the occupant is afraid to use the stairs. Poor lighting or tricky corners become obstacles that are too dangerous to navigate. Bathrooms can also be very risky places for someone with mobility issues. People who live in such an environment often feel trapped in their own house, unable to utilize the resources that were once easily at their disposal.

Depression

Clinical depression is very common among older adults. Depression has traditionally been diagnosed through a specific set of criteria established by *The Diagnostic and Statistical Manual of Mental Disorders* (DSM), now in its fifth edition. The DSM-V manual defines depression as a period of at least two weeks in which a depressed mood is accompanied by four of eight criteria: sleep problems, change in appetite, overwhelming feelings of guilt or hopelessness, loss of energy, loss of interest in previously pleasurable activities, poor concentration, hyperactivity or significant slowing of activity, or suicidal thoughts. The problem with these criteria for older adults is that issues like getting less sleep and a diminishing appetite may occur as part of the normal aging process or as part of another medical condition. Therefore, other depression screening tools have been developed to help identify depression in the geriatric population. (See Appendix G)

Depression can limit mobility because it has a negative impact on motivation and energy. Depressed persons often have no desire to initiate social contact, leading to increased loneliness and deeper depression. Furthermore, depression has a negative affect on most other medical conditions. Depression can impact concentration so severely that an older adult who is depressed sometimes appears to have dementia. The memory loss and thinking problems that can occur with depression are known as "pseudo-dementia." Dementia cannot be formally diagnosed until depression has been ruled out.

Promoting Mobility

It is possible to maintain muscle strength and mobility through some simple lifestyle habits. Proper nutrition is important for maintaining muscle and bone strength. Regular exercise is perhaps the most important factor in preserving one's mobility. Specifically, strengthening the quadriceps muscles is vitally important, a topic we'll discuss in greater detail in another chapter. It is possible to make adaptations in your home that promote safety and assist with mobility. Physical and occupational therapy may also help to preserve mobility.

Nutrition

Protein is necessary for maintaining muscle health. Foods that are high in protein include, for example, nuts, eggs, peanut butter, and meats. For various reasons, older adults sometimes have difficulty including enough protein in their diets. People who survive on a "tea and toast" diet develop vitamin deficiencies and protein malnutrition. This puts them at risk for anemia, neuropathies, and severe muscle weakness.

Anemia is another cause of weakness that can limit mobility. People who are anemic generally have less energy, and they cannot tolerate exercise as well due to poor oxygen delivery to muscle tissue. There are many causes of anemia, but the most common is probably iron deficiency. Iron plays a key role in helping hemoglobin transport oxygen throughout the body. Most older adults can benefit from an iron supplement. The main side effect of iron pills is constipation, so if your doctor suggests iron supplements, it may be wise to also take a daily stool softener. Vitamin B12 and folic acid deficiency can also cause anemia. Talk to your doctor about whether or not you should have your B12 and folic acid levels checked.

Exercise

I cannot emphasize enough the importance of establishing a regular exercise program. Our muscles and bones depend on regular use in order to maintain their vitality. The one hour per day of strenuous exercise recommended by the IOM is a noble goal, but I know few people who can practically implement this recommendation. However, thirty minutes of aerobic exercise four days per week is an excellent goal to set. Your workout routine should also include some component of weight bearing for reasons previously mentioned.

Quadriceps

The quadriceps muscles sit on the front of the thigh and connect the hip joint to the kneecap. This large set of muscles is perhaps the most important for preserving mobility. These are the muscles we use primarily to stand up and sit down. The quadriceps help us with walking and balance. They support the knee joint and protect against the development of arthritis in the knee. They also are one of the first muscle groups to atrophy once we are immobilized. Maintaining quadriceps strength is a key component to preventing the need for nursing home care.

Several simple exercises exist for strengthening the quadriceps. These exercises should be performed every day, preferably several times per day. They are easy to perform while lying in your bed. Do them when you wake up and before you go to sleep. Take time during the day to lie down and perform a set of these exercises. If you finish your repetitions and then decide to take a nap, there's nothing wrong with that. Be proud that you took time to promote your muscle health and mobility. The exercises are illustrated and explained in greater detail in Appendix B.

Household adaptations

For those with mobility difficulties, more and more products are being developed to assist with daily activities in the home. Chair lifts can assist with climbing stairs. Grab bars and slip-free shower mats can make the bathroom a much safer place. Occupational health companies can come to your home and make formal recommendations regarding safety and mobility issues. Your physician can write a prescription for such an evaluation. Home health companies can then help you equip your home so you can remain there as long as possible in the face of declining mobility

Physical and Occupational Therapy

Physical therapy and occupational therapy are excellent resources for those who need assistance with strength, balance, and mobility issues. Physical therapy is a discipline that encourages general rehabilitation by working to improve range of motion, muscle strength, balance, and joint pain. Occupational therapy focuses on specific activities important to daily function like grasping utensils, climbing stairs, or transferring from bed to chair. Many medical plans will cover both types of therapy services, specifically following an injury or other medical event. Physical therapists can come to your home if necessary. Enlisting the help of physical and occupational therapists, particularly if there is a significant decline in mobility, can be very helpful in getting you back on the right track.

Stay in Motion

Maintaining independent mobility is a key component of your body's investment strategy. Put yourself on a reasonable, regular exercise program. Make your quadriceps muscles strong. If you do nothing else during the day, spend a few minutes exercising your quadriceps. This simple action is like putting a few dollars into a stock that is just about to skyrocket in value. Obtain a home safety evaluation if you are concerned about risks within your home. Ask your physician to order a physical or occupational therapy evaluation so that risks in your home may be identified and ameliorated. You may need to pay for some of these assessments yourself, depending on your health insurance plan, but the costs are well worth it. These simple steps are strategic investments in your future independence. Start investing today.

ACTION STEPS

- Establish 4 day per week exercise routine
- Daily quadriceps exercises (appendix B)
- Arrange for a home safety/mobility evaluation

CHAPTER FOUR

WHEN YOU GOTTA GO, YOU GOTTA BE ABLE TO GET THERE!

Nancy, age eighty-two, lives alone in the home where she and her husband Donald raised their four children. Nancy had a stroke when she was seventy-five that left her partially blind and required her to walk with a cane. Donald was relatively healthy and managed the driving, cooking, and finances. When Donald died from a sudden heart attack, the family knew that Nancy would have difficulty caring for herself at home. Her daughter Lisa decided to move in with her for a while to help Nancy get used to being on her own.

Initially things went fairly well. Lisa was able to manage the shopping and housekeeping, and with the help of her siblings, got Nancy's finances in order. She arranged for meals to be delivered several times during the week through the local Department of Senior Services. Lisa was able to leave Nancy alone for several hours at a time, but she often returned to find that her mother had wet her clothes from urinary leakage.

Nancy said she just "didn't get enough warning" to get to the bathroom on time, and she needed help changing her pants because she was too worried about falling.

When they visited Nancy's doctor, they were told that Nancy had urge incontinence, a common condition among older adults. The physician prescribed a medication to help with the symptoms, but the side effects of dry mouth and dizziness upon standing were intolerable. The episodes of urinary leakage became more frequent, and Lisa began sleeping in the same room with Nancy because she would get up so frequently during the night and needed help making it safely to and from the bathroom.

The emotional and physical toll on the family began to rise. Lisa had read somewhere that urge incontinence could be helped by using the toilet every two hours, but getting Nancy back and forth to the bathroom that often became too much for one person to handle. It became necessary for Nancy to use adult diapers, and changing them was a difficult and embarrassing ordeal for the whole family. Nancy began to suffer from depression.

Lisa had never planned to live permanently with her mother, and her other siblings lived too far away to be able to help consistently. Lisa looked into hiring live-in caregivers, but the costs were significantly more than she anticipated, and the process of finding someone that both she and her mom trusted was difficult. Nancy was very uncertain about having someone unknown to the family move into her home permanently. When Nancy was hospitalized for a severe urinary tract infection, the doctor suggested that she be discharged to a nursing home for a little while to receive physical therapy and "get back on her feet." Lisa agreed, but after several weeks, Nancy still required significant help with toileting. Lisa began to wonder if her mother would ever be able to come home again.

Incontinence

The ability to use the bathroom is a key factor in keeping one's independence. Several steps are involved when your body feels the need to find the nearest restroom. First, our bodies must be able to tell us when it is "time to go." The urge created by the nerves in the bladder or rectum is our early warning sign that action is needed. The longer this lasts, the stronger the urge becomes. Next, our bodies start to expel waste by contracting certain muscles. Third, we must be able to hold in the waste until an opportune time for voiding presents itself. Finally, once we have made our way to the bathroom, we must be able to voluntarily expel the waste. A failure at any one of these steps will contribute to incontinence.

For those who suffer from incontinence, loss of bowel or bladder function often becomes the key factor that takes away their independence. Incontinence falls into two broad categories: urinary incontinence and fecal incontinence. Urinary incontinence is far more common and will be the focus of this chapter. It can be separated into four distinct categories: urge incontinence, stress incontinence, overflow incontinence, and functional incontinence. Each category has its own causes, symptoms, and preventive measures. To understand each type of incontinence, we must first understand what is actually going on inside the bladder during normal function.

Anatomy of Incontinence

The urinary bladder sits below the intestines and rests on the pubic bone. In order to understand how the bladder works, picture an upside-down balloon. The round portion of the balloon is the storage area for the urine. The kidneys clean the blood and send the waste products to the bladder via two tubes called the ureters. The top, or fundus, of the bladder is surrounded by a layer of muscle called the detrusor muscles. These muscles stretch as the bladder fills, and once they reach a certain length, they automatically contract. This is a reflex function of the nervous system and cannot be controlled voluntarily. The balloon then squeezes down and attempts to empty itself. If you've ever been stuck in traffic after having a large cup of coffee or bottle of water, you know what this feels like. It's not comfortable!

What prevents you from urinating on yourself while you're looking for that next exit ramp is the ring of muscles surrounding the neck of the bladder. These muscles encircle the stem of the upside-down balloon and tighten, closing off the bladder until you reach the bathroom. This ring of muscles is known as the urinary sphincter and is voluntarily controlled by the brain – that's why you can bypass that dirty-looking gas station in favor of a cleaner restaurant down the block ... you just flex those sphincter muscles and hope the stall is not occupied when you get to your preferred destination.

Incontinence can occur when either set of these muscles malfunction. Overflow incontinence tends to occur when the automatic response of the detrusor muscles fails to trigger timely emptying of the bladder. Stress incontinence occurs when the sphincter fails to release the urine at the appropriate time. Urge incontinence occurs when these two important functions – that of the urinary sphincter and the detrusor muscles – are not coordinated properly. Functional incontinence results from other factors in the setting of a relatively healthy bladder. A detailed explanation of each category of incontinence follows.

Consequences of Incontinence

Why is continence so important in maintaining independence? Loss of bladder function makes us dependent on others for several reasons. Incontinence is very difficult for patients and families to manage at home. Unlike losing the ability to feed, bathe, or dress, losing the ability to go the bathroom or "void" is a continuous, sometimes hourly issue that does not provide a break, even at night. It is a difficult problem to mask. It often leads to social isolation and contributes to depression.

A major problem with incontinence is, simply, it makes a mess. No one likes cleaning up excrement. There is odor, contamination, and worst of all, embarrassment. New parents may complain about having to change their infant's diapers, but ultimately parents change their baby's diapers because that's what new parents expect to do in their role as a mother or father.

On the other hand, most adult children do not expect that one day they will be changing their parents' diapers. Nor do parents expect that they may one day need help using the bathroom. I remember saying jokingly to my baby girl as I changed one of her particularly offensive diapers, "That's OK, honey. You might be changing me someday." That may be true, but when the reality of that situation strikes a family, it is no joking matter. The emotional strain alone is often enough to lead patients and families to wonder if a nursing home is a better option for someone with persistent incontinence problems.

Social isolation is another key consequence of incontinence. Many seniors who suffer from incontinence become increasingly afraid to engage in outside activities for fear of having an embarrassing accident. It becomes an easy choice to simply remain home where the problem can be contained and hidden. This leads to a more sedentary existence, contributing to loss of muscle strength and further problems in being able to reach the bathroom on time. It becomes a vicious cycle and the social isolation leads to depression, which has been proven to have a negative impact on seemingly unrelated medical conditions.

In order to understand how incontinence problems can be prevented, we must take a closer look at each type of incontinence.

Stress incontinence

Cause

Stress incontinence occurs when the muscles in the urinary sphincter lose their ability to tighten properly. Remember, these are the muscles that keep the bladder closed until we are ready to empty the bladder. In stress incontinence, urine leaks out whenever stress is applied to the bladder. Stressors include coughing, a good laugh, or even the force of gravity when standing up quickly. I've had many a good laugh with friends where "I laughed so hard I thought I would pee my pants." For those with stress incontinence, even a chuckle can turn that phrase into a reality.

Stress incontinence is more common in women for two primary reasons. First, since the length of a woman's urinary tract is shorter than a man's, there are fewer muscles present to control the outflow of urine. Men have a little more length to work with when it comes to stopping a sudden, unexpected exit of urine. Second, for women who have experienced both the joy and pain of vaginal childbirth, the pressure applied to the genitourinary region can damage the surrounding muscles and result in some loss of function. If the birth was particularly traumatic and required surgical repair, even more functional loss can occur. Scarred muscles, even when completely healed, are never as strong as they were in their original condition.

Women also tend to undergo more surgeries in the genitourinary region. Surgical manipulation of the area inevitably causes some scarring that can contribute to stress incontinence. Those who have undergone vaginal hysterectomy may experience this. Some women have what it known as bladder prolapse, when the sling of muscles supporting the bladder weakens and the bladder actually drops down toward the opening of the urethra. This can be surgically repaired, but stress incontinence can result.

Prevention and Treatment

Stress incontinence is generally easier to deal with than the other types of incontinence. Episodes become predictable as one quickly learns what types of events will trigger a leak. You can develop strategies to accommodate these triggers. Some of my patients tell me that they always stand up slowly to avoid a sudden leak. One woman revealed that she never drinks water before going out with her girlfriends because she knows she is due for a night of hearty laughter!

Adaptation to declining bodily function is sometimes the key to maintaining independence, but this approach does not directly address the problem. Instead, what one can do to address the source of stress incontinence is an exercise known as the Kegel. Named for Dr. Arnold Kegel, this exercise will strengthen your urinary sphincter and allow you to better control your urge to urinate. This exercise is key to maintain your independence and cannot be overemphasized.

The best way to describe a Kegel exercise is this: pucker your anus like you are holding in gas. This action will flex the urinary sphincter. Another way to practice flexing this muscle is to stop your flow of urine mid-stream. Hold this flexion for five to ten seconds and release. Do this over and over throughout the day. I have some patients who do Kegels every time they walk under a doorway. Some people do 10-20 Kegels each time they sit at a red light. You may be practicing them right now as you read. Keep it up! A strong urinary sphincter is one of the keys to holding on to your independence.

If the problem persists, surgeries can be performed by a urologist or urogynecologist that will reinforce the sphincter muscles. Of all types of incontinence, surgery is most helpful for stress incontinence. This is usually called "bladder sling" surgery, and doctors can use mesh tape or your own ligaments and muscles to strengthen the outlet.

Urge Incontinence

Cause

Urge incontinence occurs when the detrusor muscles on the fundus of the bladder become hyperactive. Remember our balloon analogy? The detrusor muscles are supposed to contract only when the balloon becomes stretched and full. In urge incontinence, the muscles may squeeze too early or for too long. These muscle spasms can occur spontaneously, but often they are triggered by anything that reminds the brain of a trip to the bathroom. Some people experience spasms when their feet first hit the floor in the morning. Others feel the spasms as they fumble to put their keys in the front door, rushing to get inside to use the bathroom.

When the bladder muscles contract in order to push out the urine, the pressure on the urinary sphincter increases. It is possible to flex the sphincter and "hold it" for a period of time, but often times, the combination of the strong pressure from the muscle spasm pushing down on the weakened muscles of the urinary sphincter allows leakage to occur.

Prevention and Treatment

Flexing the urinary sphincter will stop the flow of urine temporarily. The mistake many people make at that crucial point is trying to run to a toilet during a spasm. Most people cannot concentrate on getting to the bathroom quickly while also flexing their urinary sphincter at the same time. What ends up happening is your concentration on getting to the bathroom as quickly as possible overtakes your concentration to flex your urinary sphincter. As a result, your sphincter muscles relax and urine leaks out.

What most people do not realize is that the muscles spasms will pass after about 20 seconds. The best thing to do when feeling the "urge" is to stop running or, if you're walking, slow down and pause. Focus on holding in that urine and fighting off that spasm until the pressure begins to release. The pressure on your sphincter will then have decreased enough to allow you to walk to the nearest bathroom where you can then relieve your bladder.

Timed Toileting

My dad used to tell me to always keep at least ¼ tank of gas in the car during winter so it would be sure to start on those cold mornings. The opposite principle applies here. A key to preventing urge incontinence is to keep your bladder at least half empty at all times. The best way to achieve this is through timed toileting. Waiting until the bladder is full is a recipe for disaster. By that time, the spasms will be so strong and the pressure on the sphincter so great that an incontinence episode is nearly inevitable. Instead, put yourself on a schedule where you urinate every 2-3 hours while awake so that your bladder is never more than half full. This will help prevent trigger muscle spasms.

Medications

Certain medications will reduce the muscle tone of the bladder and reduce spasms; they are known as *anti-spasmodics,* and while they will work effectively for some people, they will not always work for others. There are several medications in this class, so it is often a process of trial and error before finding one that will work for you.

One significant problem with anti-spasmodics, however, is their side effects. Dry mouth and dizziness are two common complaints. Another problem is that these medicines can exacerbate dementia or confusion. Anti-spasmodic medications are also *anti-cholinergic* and block acetylcholine, a chemical that triggers muscle contractions in the bladder. For someone with dementia, blocking acetylcholine can interfere with mental status and actually worsen cognitive function. That being said, these medications have helped many people better manage their incontinence. I encourage you to explore this option with your personal physician.

Overflow Incontinence

Cause

Certain medical conditions can cause a loss of sensation in the bladder or a loss of the detrusor muscles' ability to contract once the bladder is full. Neuropathy that results from diabetes is a common cause of this condition. The consequence is a bladder that fills and fills but does not trigger or warn its owner that the bladder needs to be emptied. Eventually, the bladder cannot hold any more urine and it begins to spill out. This frequently will occur at night, and patients with this condition often wake up having wet the bed.

Prevention and Treatment

The best preventive measure for overflow incontinence is timed toileting. Use the bathroom every 2-3 hours during the day to ensure it never becomes full. Drink enough water during the day, but stop drinking two to three hours before bed time. It may be necessary to wake up at least once during the night in order to empty your bladder. Patients with diabetes should maximize their blood sugar control in order to prevent neuropathy from occurring in the first place.

Functional Incontinence

Cause

We have talked about three different types of incontinence, all of them resulting from a compromised set of detrusor muscles and/or urinary spinchter. However, your bladder control may be healthy and normal, but limited or impaired mobility makes it difficult for you to get to and from the bathroom. This leads to a condition known as functional incontinence. It is a devastating consequence of immobility, as discussed in the chapter on mobility. Functional incontinence can affect bowel and bladder control. It often leads to embarrassment, frustration, and depression. People with functional incontinence often become socially isolated because they fear having an incontinence episode in public.

Prevention

Maintaining mobility is the key to preventing functional incontinence. Tips for staying mobile can be found in the chapter on mobility.

For the Men: Prostate Problems

A major cause of incontinence in men is the condition known as benign prostatic hypertrophy (BPH). The prostate is an organ that rests in the pelvis and secretes some of the components of semen. It surrounds the urinary tube that leads out of the bladder known as the urethra. Many men experience enlargement of the prostate as they age. This increased size will press on the urethra as the prostate grows. Visualize a large straw or hose running through the middle of a donut. If the donut grows in size, it begins to press on the hose and causes it to narrow. As the urethra shrinks, the pressure makes it feel like the bladder needs to be emptied, even though it may not be full at all. The narrowing of the urethra makes it difficult to start the urine stream. It also makes it difficult for the urine to empty completely, making you feel like you have to go to the bathroom more frequently. This can lead to leaking episodes if urge incontinence or a weak urinary sphincter is already present.

Kegel exercises and timed toileting, as outlined above, will help with this problem. It is very important that men have their prostate examined regularly by a physician. A simple physical exam will diagnose an enlarged prostate most of the time. Most men with enlarged prostates have BPH, a benign condition, but some will have cancer. Some debate exists about the need for surveillance of prostate cancer among men. The blood test known as PSA is the current screening tool used to identify men with prostate cancer. Consult with your physician for his or her recommendation on the best method for prostate cancer surveillance. Medications exist that can help shrink the prostate. In more severe cases, surgery can be performed to reduce the size of the prostate or to open up the urethra. Talk to your doctor about these options.

Conclusion

Incontinence is a common problem that can become a major contributor to the need for nursing home care. Understanding the main causes of incontinence is important to knowing your own specific risk factors for developing the problem. Once the problem begins, it is also important to know the source so that preventive action can be taken. The simple steps outlined in this chapter will help anyone at any stage of life reduce their chances of requiring assistance with toileting. Those who implement these steps to avoid incontinence will dramatically reduce their odds of ending up in a nursing home.

ACTION STEPS

- Risk assessment for incontinence (appendix C)
- Daily kegel exercises
- Talk to your doctor about incontinence (he or she may not bring it up!)
- Talk to your family, health advocate, caregiver, or close confidant about incontinence
- If you are a man, have a prostate exam yearly

CHAPTER FIVE

THE HIP BONE'S CONNECTED TO YOUR VITALITY

Bill, age seventy-seven, lived in a two bedroom condo that he and his wife Claire bought when the last of their three children moved out. After Claire died three years ago, Bill kept up the condo as best as he could, with occasional help from his son, Jim, who lived nearby. His daughters, Kim and Karen, lived out of town but would usually visit on weekends and holidays. Bill had osteoporosis, and his worsening posture made it more and more difficult to move about.

One day, Bill experienced a sharp pain in his back while walking down the stairs. He went to his doctor and was diagnosed with a compression fracture in his lumbar spine. The doctor prescribed pain medication, and she explained that compression fractures require 6-8 weeks to heal. Bill did not like taking the pain medicine because it made him "woozy", but the pain was so intense that he often had difficulty even standing up.

Bill's family rallied around him. Jim, Karen and Kim figured out a plan to split time staying with Bill since he was barely able to get back and forth to the bathroom without help. At first, they managed, but Bill's pain was not improving as quickly as everyone had hoped. One night, while Kim was staying over, the pain was so intense that she called 911 and Bill was seen in the ER. He was admitted to the hospital for pain control and underwent vertebroplasty, a procedure in which a cement-like substance is injected into the vertebrae to re-expand the bone and help with the pain. Bill's pain improved, but he continued to have mobility problems. He was moved to a nursing home so he could undergo a physical therapy program to recover from the surgery. After several weeks, he still was not able to safely walk without assistance, and Bill's family began to wonder if staying at the nursing home long term might be the best option for everyone involved.

Bone Strength

Add healthy bones to the strong muscles you read about in Chapter 3, and you have the key ingredients for holding on to your independence. No matter how strong your muscles, having unhealthy bones will drastically increase your risk of moving to a nursing home. The two main bone-related causes of mobility loss are pain and fractures.

How Our Bones Are Made

Our bones are designed to withstand tremendous forces through the course of our lives. They are engineered to hold your skeleton upright, while also maintaining the ability to absorb the shocks related to transporting you from place to place. If your skeleton was too malleable, it could not hold your form. If it was solid and dense, your bones would snap like a twig from blunt force. The bone's interior design is what adapts it for mobility, and it is the key to maintaining bone health.

The firm exterior shafts of the long bones like the femur (thigh bone) house an intricate latticework of bony material. Multiple spicules of bone, called trabeculae, criss-cross throughout the interior. These trabeculae intersect at the perfect angles to provide the strong support for the varying forces applied to the bone, while allowing the bone to remain lightweight for ease of movement.

How does your body know how to engineer the blueprint for this interior structure? Bones remodel themselves based on the pressures they are asked to endure. Two types of cells are responsible for this process. *Osteoclasts* reabsorb old bone, and *osteoblasts* lay down new bone. Depending on the angle and amount of force applied to the bone, this process will adapt accordingly. Bones that are required to withstand increasing forces will ramp up their production of trabeculae, reinforcing the areas of the bone that are under the greatest stress. This process continues 24 hours a day, 7 days a week, and your entire skeleton is replaced about once every seven years.

When you are young and growing, the osteoblasts lay down new bone at a faster pace than the osteoclasts remove it. This is called bone acquisition, and it lasts until around the age of 28 when peak bone mass is achieved. Thereafter, the osteoblasts and osteoclasts keep pace with each other, but as you age, the osteoclasts begin to break down bone faster than the osteoblasts can replace it, and you start to lose bone density.

BMD is Key

Doctors measure the strength of your bones with a test called the bone mineral density (BMD) test. This test is recommended for all women over the age of 65 and should begin at the age of 60 in women with risk factors for osteoporosis, the condition causing thinning of the bones that often leads to fractures (see below). The BMD test is performed with an instrument called the dual-energy X-ray absorptiometer (DXA). This is why you will sometimes hear the BMD test referred to as a "DEXA scan."

The BMD measures the density of bone in two locations: the hip and the spine. Patients receive a number called the "T-score" which compares their bone density to a healthy, thirty-year old person of the same gender and ethnicity. The T-score is used in postmenopausal women and men over 50. The scale is a negative scale, so it can be a bit confusing. The theoretical thirty-year old to whom your bones are being compared would have a score of 0.0. Your score will be a negative number, and a T-score between 0.0 and -1.0 is considered normal. Scores between -1.0 and -2.5 put you in the classification of osteopenia, which indicates that thinning of the bones has begun but fracture risk is not high. Any score below -2.5 is considered osteoporosis. As expected, osteoporosis in the hip indicates a high risk of hip fracture, and osteoporosis found in the spine indicates a high risk of spinal fractures. Other bones are usually not measured as fractures at other sites are much less common.

Only those with a high risk of osteoporosis would undergo a BMD test. Men under 50, children, and premenopausal women receive a different score. They receive a Z-score, which is the number of standard deviations that the patient's bone density differs from a healthy person of the same age, gender, and ethnicity. As with the T-score, the lower the Z-score, the higher the risk for osteoporotic fracture.

Preventing Osteoporosis

Osteoporosis is the single biggest risk factor for a major, debilitating fracture. According to the World Health Organization, an average-sized 70 year-old woman with a T-score of -3.0 has a one in four chance of having a major osteoporotic fracture within 10 years. If this same woman lowers her T-score to -1.0, her risk is cut in half. Hip fractures are one of the leading causes of nursing home placement. Most can be repaired surgically, but the subsequent rehabilitation requires several weeks of intense physical therapy. For those who are already debilitated from other chronic illnesses, those several weeks can turn into a lifetime. In fact, people over 70 who fracture their hip have a 25% chance of dying within one year.

Bones need several things to maintain their strength. Like any engineering project, the bones need a building process, raw materials for the project, and the motivation to build. We've already talked about the process, and thankfully that was taken care of for us already through the inner programming of the osteoblasts and osteoclasts. All we need to do is provide our bodies with the raw materials and the motivation to do its work.

Store up raw materials

The key materials for bone remodeling are calcium, phosphorous, and vitamin D. Calcium is the most important building block for bone health. Its importance cannot be overemphasized. Over ninety-five percent of the calcium in our bodies resides in our bones. The primary source of calcium is through the diet, so getting enough on a daily basis is essential. The following table outlines the recommended amount you should ingest each day.

Calcium can be found in many food sources, such as dairy products and green leafy vegetables. However, many people simply do not get enough in their diet and need to take a supplement. Our gastrointestinal (GI) or digestive tract cannot absorb more than 500mg of calcium at a time, so many calcium formulations are made as 500mg tablets that should be taken three times per day if you require 1500mg per day. Many formulations also contain vitamin D, another key component for healthy bones.

Vitamin D does several things related to your bones' health. First, it assists the body's absorption of calcium and phosphorus in the GI tract. You cannot absorb enough calcium without enough vitamin D. Second, vitamin D helps regulate the parathyroid gland, a gland in the throat that controls calcium levels in the bones and bloodstream. When blood calcium levels are low, this gland secretes parathyroid hormone (PTH), which causes the osteoclasts (the type of bone cells that reabsorbs old bone) to increase their activity and release calcium from the bone into the bloodstream. Active vitamin D can turn off PTH if too much calcium is being reabsorbed from the bones. Third, vitamin D can halt the kidney from excreting too much calcium and phosphorus through the urine.

Phosphorus also assists with bone formation, but the amounts needed in the body are much smaller and usually are acquired through a balanced diet. People with kidney disease often need to take a phosphorus supplement because their kidneys excrete too much phosphorus. Otherwise, the ingestion and metabolism of phosphorus is fairly automatic and will not require much of your attention as you strive to maintain your independence.

Motivate Your Osteoblasts

Now that you have your building blocks, your body needs some motivation. You can give it this motivation through exercise. As described above, the stresses placed on the bones have a direct impact on the activity of the osteoblasts and osteoclasts. The more you demand of your bones, the more they will respond. Osteoporosis is a disease of either a lack of building blocks (calcium and vitamin D) or a lack of exercise, or both. An exercise program that will give the bones some healthy stress is a key to reducing fracture risk.

Walking or running will provide the bones with the necessary impact to motivate your osteoblasts. It may be helpful to carry small weights or use ankle weights to provide some additional stress. Many people are unable to run or even perform high impact walking due to joint pains and arthritis. If this is the case for you, weightlifting is another activity that provides some bone stress that tends not to damage the joints. Talk with your doctor about getting started on a healthy exercise regimen.

Medications

Once osteoporosis sets in, most doctors will recommend a medication called a bisphosphonate. These medications assist the body in laying down new bone. They do not work if there is not enough calcium, and their effect is also enhanced by high impact exercise. Many of these drugs can be taken once per week, and some can be taken once per month. Bisphosphonates may cause acid reflux and, therefore, must be taken in a very specific way (for example, it is recommended that you not lie down for at least thirty minutes after having taken the medication). Some patients simply cannot tolerate these medicines due to the side effects. For those who can, the drugs have been shown in many studies to reduce fracture risk and help rebuild osteoporotic bone.

Prevention is Key

Some falls are impossible to avoid. As you age, your risk of falling increases. Take the necessary steps to strengthen your bones and guard against a major fracture. Someone with strong bones may end up with nothing more than a bruised backside, while those who are unprepared could see a simple slip off the back stoop turn into a trip to the hospital, a long rehabilitation, and perhaps a permanent residence in a long-term care facility. Don't let that slip off the stoop be your last experience in your treasured home.

ACTION STEPS

- Ensure adequate calcium and vitamin D intake (appendix D)
- Have a BMD test if you are in a high risk group (appendix E)
- Weight bearing exercise plan at least twice per week

CHAPTER SIX

KEEP THE PIPES CLEAN

What does it mean to be "healthy?" One of the first things we think of is cardiovascular fitness. The image of a healthy human being usually involves a person who can run long distances, climb mountains, and persevere through intense demands on the body. This type of fitness is only possible with good cardiovascular health. To most people, "cardiovascular" health is synonymous with heart health. They are only half right.

Cardiovascular Health: What's the Big Deal?

"Cardio-" does indeed mean "heart," and keeping our heart healthy is extremely important. However, we sometimes forget about the "-vascular" part of "cardiovascular." Vascular means "related to the blood vessels," and it's not just the blood vessels in our heart that we need to care for. The arteries that carry oxygen-rich blood to organs throughout the body, and the veins that return the blood to our heart and lungs for a refill of oxygen, must be functioning properly if we are to maintain independence. The regions of the body that are particularly sensitive to good vascular health are the brain, the kidneys, the heart, and the extremities. Before examining each of these systems and their contribution to independence, we will explore the blood vessel itself.

General Vascular Health

The system of blood vessels that course through the body continually supplies organ tissues with oxygen. These arteries, veins, and capillaries are uniquely designed to maintain a continual flow of vital nutrients to all parts of our being. Large arteries, like the aorta that leads out of the left side of the heart, and the iliac arteries that branch off the aorta in the lower abdomen and travel to the legs, have thick, durable walls and wide open space. The aorta is about the diameter of a garden hose. Large amounts of blood can rush through these large vessels at high pressure and velocity. As the arteries traverse to their intended destination, they continue to branch, and they become more narrow and more delicate. The blood's rate of travel declines sharply, and by the time the blood cells reach the organs, they are slowly drifting through a nest of tiny capillaries, similar to vacationers who drift on inner tubes at a recreational water park's "lazy river." These vessels are so small that it would take ten of them stacked together to equal the thickness of a human hair.

Here in the capillaries, the oxygen carried by the red blood cells diffuses into the tissues, delivering a key component for the energy reactions that keep cells alive and functioning. The blood cells now begin their reverse course through the veins, where they will re-enter the heart and pump quickly through the lungs, via the pulmonary circulation, so they can refill with oxygen.

This entire process of traveling out of the heart, to the organs, back to the heart, and through the lungs, takes the average blood cell about twenty seconds. Your entire blood supply circulates through the vascular system over 4000 times per day.

Every Vessel Has a Fragile Lining

The inside of your blood vessels are coated with a unique lining called the endothelium. This lining allows the blood to travel smoothly throughout the circulatory system, and it regulates the passage of blood cells and fluid into and out of the blood vessels from the adjacent tissues. The endothelial cells can sense the smallest changes in pressure, and they send signals to the muscles that line the blood vessels. These muscles are under autonomic control, meaning that you don't have to consciously commend them to contract or relax. If, for example, an organ is injured and needs a sudden infusion of blood for oxygen and inflammatory cells that promote healing, the muscles lining the vessels will contract, causing narrowing of the vessel, or vasoconstriction. This will force the blood to travel faster to the area in need. When an area of the body is saturated with oxygen, the muscles in the vessel walls will relax, causing the vessels to open wider, or dilate, and reducing the flow. This process is occurring continually under the supervision of the autonomic nervous system, an intricate and unconscious signaling operation that is responsible for our "fight or flight" response. In most parts of the body, when we are relaxed, the blood vessels dilate, and when we are under stress, they contract, an important point to remember when we discuss blood pressure control later in the chapter.

The endothelial cells lining the blood vessel walls are exquisitely sensitive to something called oxidative stress. Oxidative stress occurs when certain proteins and other substance break down in the body as part of their natural life cycle. Oxidation is sped up in the setting of inflammation. The side products of oxidation are particles called "free radicals" which do damage to the endothelial tissue. This results in scarring, leading to the formation of a plaque, or a raised patch on the lining of the vessel. These plaques are mostly made up of cholesterol, an essential component of many of the membranes in our body. By forming a plaque, the body is making a sort of scab on the inside of the blood vessel to cover the damage created by the chemical reactions related to oxidation. Plenty of medical research over the past two decades has gone into reducing oxidative stress within the body, and this is why foods containing antioxidants are touted as helping to prevent the effects of aging.

Damage to the endothelial lining of our vessels also occurs due to pressure. The autonomic nervous system, by the process described above, maintains a steady pressure throughout our vascular system. The body tries to regulate the pressure so it is high enough to deliver sufficient oxygen and nutrients to the organs, but not too high so as to cause damage. As you would expect, smaller, more fragile blood vessels are especially sensitive to changes in pressure. If a blood vessel has to endure a continually high level of internal pressure, the endothelial cells lining the vessel are damaged, and plaques begin to form, just as they do under oxidative stress.

The Straight and Narrow Road Isn't Always Healthy

Plaque formation along the lining of a blood vessel is known as atherosclerosis. The result is a narrowed tube that is much less efficient at delivering blood to its destination. The body will often try to compensate for the poor delivery by increasing the pressure through the narrow tube, and it may work for a while, but the increased pressure also adds to the problem. The body can also find ways around a clogged artery by redirecting the circulation through adjacent vessels known as collateral arteries. We can even grow new arteries to detour around a blockage through a process known as neovascularization. Unfortunately, this process produces only a second rate delivery system that is even more susceptible to the same damaging forces that caused the original blockage.

Now that you understand the basics of blood vessel function and why they narrow, let us examine the effects that vascular disease can have on some organ systems that are essential to functional independence.

Heart

If you live into your seventies, your heart will beat over 2.5 billion times. The cardiac muscle in the heart is uniquely designed to produce the same amount of force as skeletal muscles, like in the arms and legs, but with a continuous, unconscious rhythm, like the autonomic muscles lining the blood vessels and gastrointestinal tract. Heart muscle needs a continual flow of oxygen, supplied by the coronary arteries that line the outside of the heart. These small vessels take oxygen-rich blood straight from the left ventricle, the largest chamber of the heart, and into the heart muscles.

When these coronary arteries become narrowed via the processes already discussed, doctors will assign the diagnosis of coronary artery disease (CAD), commonly known as heart disease. As described above, the body can compensate for a blockage in a coronary artery through collateral circulation and neovascularization. In fact, three or four major arteries can narrow by 80-90%, and the heart can continue to function normally for a time. All too often, the first sign of severe CAD is a heart attack, when the heart muscle is getting so little oxygen that it begins to die. When heart muscle dies, it creates intense chest pain, and even worse, the efficiency of the pump begins to fail. This becomes life-threatening, because now the heart is not able to maintain enough pressure through the vascular system to deliver oxygen to other vital organs.

If the person with CAD is lucky, they will begin to experience heart-related chest pain, or angina, long before muscle damage begins to occur, alerting them to the problem in time to intervene. Muscles that lack oxygen go into an alternative process to produce energy. This process is far less efficient and creates a toxic byproduct, lactic acid. As the lactic acid builds, the muscles send out pain signals, as any marathon runner will tell you when they "hit the wall" around mile 20 and their legs start to scream at them. This same phenomenon can occur in the heart, which is why people with CAD often experience chest pain with exertion. In contrast to other muscle pain, angina is usually described as "heaviness" or "pressure" rather than sharp, and any patient who speaks of chest pressure with exercise is sure to get their doctor's immediate attention and concern.

Doctors diagnose CAD with angiography, the process of inserting a catheter tube into a vein in the leg and passing it into the heart. Radiographic dye is then injected into the coronary arteries, and the images will reveal any narrowing or blockages. If the passage is not too narrow, doctors can immediately open the vessel with an inflatable balloon or by placing a mesh tube known as a stent. If the blockages are severe or multiple, bypass surgery is often required. A healthy vein is removed from the leg or another part of the body, and attached to the heart vessel above and below the blockage, creating a detour. Most people who undergo cardiac bypass have multiple blockages, which is why you often hear of triple or quadruple bypass procedures.

The sudden, gripping onset of a heart attack, the modern miracle of open heart surgeries, and the made-for-television drama of resuscitation attempts with electric shocks capture our attention and often define our image of heart disease. In reality, heart disease develops slowly and often does not result in such dramatic outcomes. Heart muscle remodels in response to poor oxygen delivery, and it sometimes grows and thickens to compensate. Thickened heart muscle is actually less efficient, and the problem exacerbates. The chambers of the heart will also dilate to try and generate more pressure to expel the blood. The culmination of these adaptive efforts leads to the condition known as congestive heart failure (CHF). CHF is a debilitating, progressive, and incurable illness that will quickly lead to a loss of independence.

Patients with CHF have hearts that do not pump efficiently. The pumping action of the heart can be measured with an ultrasound of the heart called an echocardiogram. Doctors assign a number to describe the effectiveness of the pump, called the ejection fraction. It is an estimate of the percentage of blood that actually leaves the heart with each heartbeat. Normal hearts push out 60-70% of the blood in their chambers during a contraction. People with CHF often have ejection fractions of 30-40% or lower.

The primary symptom of CHF is shortness of breath. Since the heart cannot pump the blood through the system efficiently, the fluid tends to back up into the lungs and the veins. The result is pulmonary edema, or lungs that fill with fluid, so they cannot process oxygen well or inflate and deflate comfortably. Patients especially feel this shortness of breath when they lay flat, since the fluid tracks up to the top of their lungs due to gravity. Many patients with CHF sleep sitting up in a chair because it is too uncomfortable to lie down.

Another hallmark of CHF is exertional dyspnea, or shortness of breath with any level of exertion. This is where CHF begins to rob patients of their independence. Many patients lose their ability to climb stairs, walk to the mailbox, or navigate their own home due to the intense fatigue and difficulty breathing they feel with even the smallest amount of effort. Walking across a parking lot from a car to the store becomes out of the question. The oppressive symptoms lead to isolation, and often depression, worsening the problem further.

Treatment for CHF often involves diuretic medication, which helps the body remove the excess fluid through the urine. These drugs produce frequent urination, and for those who are already on the brink of functional incontinence due to their frail nature, starting a diuretic will often push them over the edge. The CHF symptoms may improve, but the new incontinence could make it too difficult to remain at home without help. This is one example of the "rock and a hard place" scenarios that we often encounter in geriatric medicine. The combined effect of poor tolerance for exertion and increasing dependence on medications leads to more and more dependence on others for daily living. Many people with CHF must wear continuous oxygen, another limit to one's mobility. These factors make cardiac disease a leading cause of functional dependence, leading to nursing home placement.

Brain

Brain cells, or neurons, are the most sensitive cells in our body to a drop in oxygen levels. The average brain cell can survive only eight minutes without oxygen. Adequate blood flow through the brain is vital to maintaining cognitive function. The brain is full of tiny vessels that saturate the neurons with essential oxygen and nutrients. These vessels are particularly sensitive to changes in pressure. Many have sharp, ninety-degree branches that are subject to shearing forces which can create damage. When vessels in the brain become narrowed or blocked, it is known as cerebrovascular disease, one of the most common contributors to loss of independence. The most obvious consequence of cerebrovascular disease is a stroke.

A stroke, or cerebrovascular accident (CVA), occurs for two reasons. The most dramatic kind of stroke is the hemorrhagic stroke, when a blood vessel in the brain bursts and bleeds onto surrounding tissue. This causes immediate damage to the brain cells, and as the blood collects, it produces pressure with the cranial space that holds the brain. This confined space cannot tolerate even small shifts in pressure, and surrounding brain tissue begins to suffer as well. Depending on where in the brain it occurs, the hemorrhagic stroke typically causes instantaneous symptoms such as slurred speech, drooling, loss of strength on one side of the body or the other, or vision loss.

The second, and more common, type of stroke is the ischemic stroke. Ischemic strokes account for 80% of all CVA's. In this case, a blockage occurs in the blood vessels and the blood supply to an area of the brain is cut off. The brain cells begin to die, often producing symptoms similar to those in hemorrhagic stroke, as described above. Blockages can occur due to endothelial damage, or due to a phenomenon known as embolization. Tiny blood clots from other areas of the body can break off and travel to the brain, where they lodge in a capillary and interrupt the blood flow. These clots most often form in the heart, particularly among people with abnormal heart rhythms. Blood requires consistent, or laminar, flow in order to remain fluid. By design, turbulent flow triggers factors in the blood to begin to form clots. People with an irregular heartbeat known as atrial fibrillation are usually placed on blood thinners, because they are at particular risk for forming a clot in their heart that could travel to the brain and cause an ischemic stroke.

At the first sign of stroke, it is imperative to seek medical attention immediately. Surgeons can evacuate, or remove, the accumulating blood from a hemorrhagic stroke, and hence relieve the pressure and preserve sensitive brain tissue. Ischemic strokes can be treated with powerful "clotbuster" medications, which will dissolve the clot or blockage instantly and restore blood flow to the affected neurons. Once the brain cells die, the damage is often permanent, though the brain sometimes has the ability to recover function over weeks to months. This is a long process, and people with other debilitating medical conditions often do not have the endurance to undergo the intense physical therapy necessary to give the brain a chance to recuperate.

Just as heart disease does not always present with a heart attack, cerebrovascular disease does not always manifest itself as a stroke. Transient ischemic attacks (TIA), or "mini-strokes," occur when the circulation to one area of the brain is temporarily cut off and then restored. By definition, the symptoms of a TIA resolve within 24 hours. When a TIA occurs, it is a warning sign that cerebrovascular disease is present in the brain.

Cerebrovascular disease can take a toll even in the absence of strokes or TIAs. As you will learn in the chapter on brain function, the second leading cause of dementia is cerebrovascular disease. Vascular dementia occurs when the general circulation within the brain is compromised. Over time, cells throughout the brain are damaged, leading to a steady decline in global function without an obvious sign of neurologic damage. Even sensitive radiologic tests like computed tomography (CT) scans and magnetic resonance imaging (MRI) studies cannot always detect the damage that is occurring in miniscule areas across the brain. The effects on the patient's function, however, are very apparent.

The combined effect of stroke and vascular dementia may be the most common cause of nursing home placement in the

United States. Many people are not able to fully rehabilitate from a stroke, and those with paralysis on one side of the body have instantaneous need for help with their ADLs. Adaptations can be made, and physical and occupational therapists can assist patients in developing strategies for navigating their home in spite of their new deficits, but often the transition back home is impossible. In the chapter on brain function, we will see how dementia, an irreversible process, leads to nursing home placement in a majority of cases.

Kidney

The kidney is another organ that depends on adequate circulatory function. As with the heart and the brain, the circulation in the kidney consists of many small, branching blood vessels that supply oxygen and nutrients to cells that cannot survive without a consistent infusion. High blood pressure, or hypertension, does particular damage to vessels in the kidney over months and years. Next to diabetes, hypertension is the most common cause of kidney disease. Uncontrolled hypertension can destroy kidney function to the point that hemodialysis is required.

Chronic kidney disease does not have a cure, and it tends to get worse over time. As kidney disease advances, fewer and fewer medications can be used to treat other conditions like heart disease and diabetes, because the kidney is unable to clear them from the system. This leads to more rapid deterioration and increased levels of dependence. Simple infections can progress to life-threatening, overwhelming contamination of the bloodstream, or sepsis. Patients who need hemodialysis are required to visit a dialysis center for 4-5 hours, three times per week, and missing even one session could lead to hospitalization or even death. The limits on independence from kidney disease are obvious.

Extremities

Many parts of the body can compensate for poor blood flow through collateral circulation, as described above. In the extremities, and particularly the feet, there is no opportunity for detours around a blockage or compromised vessel. Peripheral arterial disease (PAD), a condition in which the blood vessels in the extremities narrow or develop blockages, can do severe damage to the legs. A telltale sign of PAD is pain in the calves that gets worse with walking or exertion. The development of this symptom should prompt a trip to the doctor. Another more common vascular condition in the legs is venous stasis, when the blood has a difficult time returning to the heart through the veins. Venous stasis develops over time as we age. Common signs are multiple varicose veins or a diffuse, purplish discoloration that evolves in front of the ankles and on the shins. The condition leads to pooling blood in the feet and legs that interferes with efficient circulation.

Poor circulation leads to the development of pain, skin ulcers, and severe infections that cannot heal. Ulcers of the foot are especially vulnerable to infection, because the lack of blood flow prohibits the delivery of white blood cells, our body's "soldier" cells that can eliminate bacteria and other invaders. In the worst cases, these ulcers can progress to gangrenous lesions that require amputation.

When a wound does not heal, it is almost always due to poor circulation. For obvious reasons, non-healing leg and foot ulcers take a major toll on independence. Pain can limit the ability to walk. Circulation can be improved with elevation of the legs, in order to improve venous return to the heart, but this also limits the patient to remaining in a bed or chair most of the time. Immobility leads to muscle atrophy, and a downward spiral begins. Infected ulcers can emit a foul odor that leads to social isolation. Many patients with a non-healing ulcer prefer to remain at home rather than face the embarrassment of presenting an ugly, painful, or smelly bandaged wound to the public. Depression is common among those with non-healing wounds.

Prevention

The marvelous thing about the cardiovascular system is that everything you do to improve the health of your blood vessels will apply to the entire body. Steps you take to improve circulation in your brain will also encourage blood flow to the extremities. Building your heart's endurance will also strengthen the kidneys. The primary factors where you can intervene to improve your vascular health are blood pressure, cholesterol, inflammation, and stress.

Blood Pressure

The vascular system must remain under pressure in order to sustain the flow of blood to vital organs. Patients who go into shock experience a sudden drop of blood pressure, and emergency response teams pour intravenous fluids and medications into these patients in order to maintain adequate blood pressure to protect the brain and other tissues from death. While an extremely low blood pressure can be life-threatening, the body can tolerate higher than normal blood pressures for months and years without obvious signs or symptoms. Even so, damage occurs that will eventually lead to significant loss of function. Over time, blood vessels that are called upon to survive in a high pressure environment will develop interior damage and scarring, leading to narrowing, blockages, and poor flow via the processes describe earlier in this chapter.

Blood pressure measurements consist of two numbers. The top number represents the systolic pressure, or the amount of pressure produced when the heart contracts and pushes blood through the system. The bottom number is the diastolic pressure and represents the phase when heart is relaxed. Over the past fifty years, there has been more research on the impact of blood pressure than almost any other aspect of health.

The research shows that people who maintain healthy blood pressures have better health outcomes across the board, but particularly in the organ systems mentioned above. For years, a reading of 120 over 80 was touted as the ultimate goal for healthy blood pressure. Recently, the 7th meeting of the Joint National Commission on Blood Pressure lowered this recommendation to 115/75, based on decades of research related to heart attacks, strokes, and kidney disease. People with blood pressures between 115/75 and 135/85 are considered to have "prehypertension" and are at higher risk for strokes and heart attacks than those with lower pressures. For every 20 point increase in the systolic pressure (top number) and every 10 point increase in the diastolic pressure (bottom number), your risk for heart attack or stroke doubles.

Over 90% of cases of hypertension fall into the category of "essential" hypertension, a form of high blood pressure that does not have any root physical cause in the body other than genetics. Hypertension does run in families, though there is not a direct genetic link that is known. There are unusual cases of hypertension caused by stenosis (narrowing) of the large arteries in the kidney, electrolyte imbalances caused by thyroid or adrenal gland problems, or tumors that secrete hormones that raise the blood pressure. Specialized testing for these conditions can be ordered by your doctor, but only if he or she suspects these conditions, or if the blood pressure is not responding to standard treatments.

Lifestyle factors play a major role in blood pressure maintenance. Unlike a machine or an engine that wears down with use, our bodies become more efficient the more we ask of them. Distance athletes like Lance Armstrong have resting blood pressures in the 80/40 range and a resting pulse of 35 beats per minute because their cardiovascular system has become highly efficient at pumping blood. Regular aerobic exercise develops this efficiency, so that even when we are not placing intense demands on the heart and blood vessels, they function at a healthier pace.

Aerobic exercise is defined as sustained activity (more than ten minutes) that achieves a target heart rate. The target heart rate can be calculated by subtracting 220 from your age if you are a man, or 226 from your age if you are a woman. An ideal practice is to participate in at least thirty minutes of aerobic exercise four days per week or more.

Have your blood pressure checked at your doctor's office on two separate occasions in order to get the most accurate results. You can check it yourself, but over the counter blood pressure monitors vary in accuracy, as do the monitors found at retails stores and pharmacies. Furthermore, blood pressure is most accurate when you are seated and resting for at least five minutes. (And you wondered why we made you sit and wait in that cold room for so long!) Anxiety can increase blood pressure, and in some people, a phenomenon called "white coat hypertension" does occur, when the reading is artificially inflated due to the stress of being at the doctor. Home blood pressure monitoring can be arranged in such cases for the most accurate result.

Another useful measure of cardiovascular health is the resting pulse. Research has shown that people with a resting pulse under 83 beats per minute have much lower rates of heart attack and stroke than those with a higher pulse. The best way to check a resting pulse is to measure it yourself when you first wake up in the morning. Before getting out of bed, take your index and middle fingers and find your pulse on your wrist or next to your throat. Count the number of beats in a minute and you have your resting pulse.

Cholesterol

The body's membranes, or thin layers that surround cells and other tissues, are partly made up of the substance cholesterol. This substance is important for your survival, but as you have heard many times, high cholesterol can also be a killer. People with increased levels of a certain type of cholesterol, the low-density lipoprotein (LDL), are also at increased risk for vascular disease. The LDL molecules float through the blood stream and deposit on the walls of the vessels, leading to gradual narrowing. Plaques form, as described previously, and these plaques can rupture suddenly, causing a 20% blockage to rapidly become an 80 or 100% blockage. This is the mechanism for many sudden heart attacks. While most people think of cholesterol deposits causing heart disease, high cholesterol can cause vascular disease anywhere in the body, but especially in the other sensitive areas we discussed: the brain, kidneys, and extremities.

Certain families have a strong genetic predisposition towards high cholesterol, and their cholesterol levels should be tested in their twenties. For the rest of us, an initial test should be performed in the thirties, and then more frequent monitoring can begin in the fifties. Regular exercise will lower cholesterol levels. Foods high in fat will increase cholesterol, but foods high in omega-3 fatty acids, like tuna and salmon, will actually reduce your LDL levels. This is especially true of certain nuts like walnuts, almonds, and pecans. Regular intake of bran will also bring down the cholesterol a few points.

For those who cannot achieve acceptable levels with lifestyle changes, there are very effective medicines for lowering cholesterol. The "statin" class of drugs can dramatically bring down LDL levels, and these medicines have been shown to reduce heart attacks and strokes significantly over the past two decades. The most common side effect of statin drugs is muscle pain. These drugs can cause a condition called rhabdomyolysis, in which the muscles begin to actually break down by chemically digesting themselves. If you are taking a statin and you experience muscle aches or pains, see your doctor.

Some people are blessed with high levels of "good" cholesterol, the high-density lipoprotein (HDL). This cholesterol can protect your heart and blood vessels better than any medicine. The LDL is best remembered as the "Lousy" cholesterol, and the HDL as the "Happy" cholesterol. A lipid panel blood test will contain levels of both the LDL and HDL, and your doctor will help you interpret the results.

Inflammation and Stress

Much current research on the cardiovascular system focuses on the effects of inflammation on the body. When the body is under attack from a foreign substance, an organism, or an injury, it naturally produces a cascade of internal cellular events in order to heal itself. Most of the time, this reaction is essential to health and can be life-saving. If your body is invaded by a potentially deadly virus or bacteria, the inflammatory response sends white blood cells to fight the intruder, releases substances toxic to cells in order to kill the unwelcome guests, and increases the pulse and blood pressure to quickly deliver these life-saving components to the correct area of the body.

Unfortunately, inflammation can occur when the body is not being threatened. Stress is the primary cause for the inflammatory state, though more research is suggesting that the ingestion of chemicals and preservatives found in the Western diet also contributes significantly to this problem. When your body is living under continual stress, it remains in a state of inflammation, causing a continual onslaught of oxidative stress to the lining of the vessels.

Stress reduction is important for all aspects of health, but especially for vascular health. You may not be able to reduce or eliminate all the stressors in your life, but you do have control over how you manage that stress. Start by taking at least fifteen minutes per day to establish a quiet thought pattern and slow your breathing. This can be accomplished by prayer, meditation, yoga, or other techniques. Learning to breath more slowly is an important strategy for reducing stress. Giving your brain a chance to reset each day allows you to release built up anxiety. Sleep is also critical to stress reduction. Discipline yourself to get seven to eight hours of sleep per night, and you will be surprised at your improved efficiency. Regular exercise is also a very effective stress reducer.

When aspirin was first introduced, it was dubbed "the wonder drug" due to its many uses. With the advent of safer and more effective pain medications, the role of aspirin has changed, but it remains important. Aspirin inhibits platelets, the cells in the blood that initiate clotting. Platelets serve an important purpose when you bleed from a cut or wound, but they can also contribute to blockages in the vessels if they are triggered by oxidative stress. Taking one aspirin per day, in either the 81mg or 325mg dose, appears to reduce the risk of heart attack and stroke for most people. It may even improve blood flow in the brain enough to reduce the risk of vascular dementia. There is a chance of gastrointestinal bleeding with regular aspirin use, so talk to your doctor about whether a daily aspirin is right for you.

A Word About Smoking

You know that smoking is bad for you. I will go one step further- smoking is *terrible* for you. You know that smoking damages your lungs. I will go another step- smoking damages your *entire body*. The chemicals contained in cigarette and cigar smoke cause tremendous damage to the lining of your blood vessels. It is the same sort of damage discussed earlier in this chapter, only the damage occurs at a faster and more reliable rate than with high cholesterol or high blood pressure. In addition to circulatory problems, many smokers have chronic obstructive pulmonary disease (COPD), also known as emphysema, an incurable lung condition that leads to shortness of breath with even light exertion. COPD is becoming one of the leading causes of death in the US. Smokers are at higher risk for heart disease, stroke, and diabetes. As a result, smoking increases your risk for ending up in a nursing home.

If you do not smoke, never start. If you do smoke, there is good news. More and more research and resources are available for people who want to quit smoking and "breath free." Talk to your doctor about your options. Making the choice to breathe free of cigarettes is the single best thing you can do for your health.

Take Care of the Pipes

Your vascular system is the literal lifeline for your vital organs. Your independence will be threatened if you do not care for your blood vessels. Congestive heart failure, kidney failure, and dementia all can develop from years of small but progressive damage that occurs when risk factors for vascular disease are not controlled. A stroke can be devastating and dramatically increases your chance of needing nursing home care. Take some simple steps today to maximize your blood flow and your chance to remain independent.

ACTION STEPS

- Measure your blood pressure and resting pulse rate
- Test your cholesterol
- Talk to your doctor about your goals for these numbers and how to achieve them
- Develop an aerobic exercise plan (30 minutes, four times per week or more)
- Eat tuna or salmon twice per week
- Add walnuts, almonds or pecans to your diet
- Incorporate fiber into your daily regimen
- Talk to your doctor about taking one aspirin per day
- Get 7-8 hours of sleep per night
- Pray, meditate, or perform another brain-calming and breath-slowing exercise for fifteen minutes or more per day
- If you smoke, talk to your doctor and make a plan to quit

IF I ONLY HAD A HEALTHY BRAIN

Mary, age sixty-seven, lived with her husband Jack, age seventy, in the house where they raised their three children. Jack and Mary were relatively healthy. Jack had high blood pressure that was controlled with medication, and Mary's low thyroid levels had been managed successfully for years with daily thyroid supplements. Jack played golf once a week, and Mary enjoyed knitting sweaters for their grandchildren. Jack paid the bills and Mary did the grocery shopping. Two of Jack and Mary's adult children lived nearby and brought the grandchildren over many Sunday afternoons.

The first sign of trouble came when Mary's daughter Julie brought her children to bake chocolate-chip cookies with grandma. The girls proudly presented the batch to the family, and they quickly noticed that the cookies tasted quite different from the usually delicious "grandma's cookies." Mary had the recipe memorized, but she wondered if she had followed it correctly this time. Her family excused Mary for being distracted by the rambunctious girls' "help." Julie said, "I can't get anything done properly when they're helping me!" and everyone had a good laugh.

Later that month, Jack noticed that the cupboards contained an abundance of flour. He asked Mary if she was planning on baking a large batch of bread, and she said "No, I must have forgotten that I bought flour the last time I was at the store." Soon, Mary began to have difficulty filling out the grocery list. Jack noticed her one day sitting at the kitchen table in tears because she could not recall what she needed to buy each week. They made an appointment with their primary doctor.

Jack related the story to the physician, who seemed especially interested in the crying spells. He diagnosed Mary with depression and explained that depression can have a profound effect on concentration and focus. He prescribed a mild antidepressant and told Jack and Mary that it would take about six weeks for the medication to take effect. He also ordered a thyroid test to make sure her levels were still in normal range. No one, including the doctor, wanted to bring up the word "dementia."

Six weeks later, Mary was crying less and her mood had improved. Her thyroid test was normal. She told the doctor that she felt better, and he gave her three months of refills on the antidepressant. Everything seemed back to normal.

Two months later, Mary left for the grocery store and did not return for three hours. Jack called her cell phone and she answered, sounding frantic. "I don't know where I am, Jack. I got lost coming home." She described some local landmarks. Jack told her to stay where she was, called his son, and they drove together to find her physically unharmed but very unnerved. Jack drove her home and they made another appointment.

This time, the doctor performed some memory tests with Mary. She scored a 23 out of 30 on the mini-mental status exam (MMSE). That sounded like a pretty good score, but the doctor informed them that a score of 23 classified Mary in the early stage of dementia. The couple was devastated and peppered the doctor with questions about what to do next. He stopped her antidepressant and ordered some tests to rule out other causes of memory problems. The tests were normal, so the doctor diagnosed Mary with Alzheimer's disease and prescribed a different medication this time, one that was designed to slow the progression of the dementia.

Nine months later, Mary's memory was worsening and it was wearing on Jack. He patiently answered her repetitive questions about the day's activities. He had taken over the grocery shopping, cooking, cleaning, and every other aspect of caring for the household. One night he awoke and did not find Mary next to him in bed. He rushed downstairs to find Mary pacing in the living room, muttering about needing to visit her mother. When he approached her, she yelled and would not let him touch her. He called his son and he came over. They didn't know what to do, so they took her to the emergency room.

Mary remained confused and combative at the ER, and she was given medication to calm her down. The doctor ran some tests and found she had a urinary tract infection and was mildly dehydrated. They admitted her to the hospital for observation and treatment of the infection. She continued to have episodes of confusion in the hospital. During her hospitalization, Mary became weak from lying in bed, and the hospital doctor recommended a short-term stay at a nursing home for some physical therapy. Mary was moved to a skilled nursing facility.

Mary's advancing dementia made it difficult for her to follow commands and participate in the therapy. Her persistent episodes of nighttime confusion prompted the staff to sedate her with medications, which also made her drowsy during the daytime, interfering further with her ability to complete the course of physical therapy. When Jack met with the nursing home staff, they questioned his ability to care for Mary at home in her current state. Long-term placement at the facility began to look inevitable.

Brain Function

The brain is the most important organ that helps us maintain our independence. In order to function independently, we rely on our brains to learn new information and to recall previously learned information. Our brains need to process language, recognize objects and their purposes, and command our bodies to carry out tasks. We must maintain the crucial cerebral skills of planning, organizing, sequencing, and abstracting, if we are to operate independently. A decline in any one of these skills threatens our independence.

Take, for example, the ability to drive a car, an activity most adults take for granted. Driving from one location to another requires the ability to learn and comprehend a planned route, or to remember a previously traveled route. We must be able to read a roadside sign and process its meaning, usually at a rapid pace. Our brains must recall the purpose of the many unlabeled instruments that operate the vehicle, like keys, steering wheel, stick shift, pedals, windshield wipers, etc. Our brains must then send commands to our muscles to manipulate these objects, often quickly, in response to the constantly changing circumstances of the road, which the brain must also process efficiently and accurately. As we are doing all these things, the brain has to think ahead to the next moves in order to get us where we are going. It's amazing that many of us can do all of this while talking on the phone, reading a map, eating breakfast, or doing all three at once (something I do not recommend!).

Aging causes a general slowing in all of these abilities. However, sometimes the functional decline of the brain happens more rapidly, affecting one or more crucial skills more severely. For example, someone who begins to lose their ability to plan ahead logically (a skill known as executive function) cannot necessarily be trusted to safely operate an automobile. The general term for the abnormal loss of brain function is cognitive impairment, and when it progresses to the point of interfering with daily function, we use the term "dementia." Dementia is one of the most important contributors to nursing home admissions in the United States.

Multiple Causes

Dementia can be caused by multiple factors. The most common cause is Alzheimer's disease. Alzheimer's is a genetic disorder that affects over 5 million Americans. We have a clear understanding of what happens to the brain in

Alzheimer's, but we don't fully understand why it happens or how to stop the process.

Alzheimer's is the result of two distinct processes. First, collections of fibers begin to form in the brain called "neurofibrillary tangles." These tangles take up space from normal brain tissue and interfere with transmission of brain signals between the neurons. (Neurons are the trillions of cells within the brain that constantly share essential information.) Second, plaques, or collections of protein, build up between brain cells and interfere with normal function. As mentioned earlier, this disturbance of the brain's normal abilities is known as cognitive impairment.

The second most common type of dementia is called vascular dementia. It is the result of circulation problems in the brain. The blood vessels in the brain are very delicate and are subject to damage from the shearing forces of blood pressure. High blood pressure predisposes these small vessels to damage along the interior walls, leading to narrowing of the vessels and impeding blood flow. This can be further exacerbated by blockages created by cholesterol deposits, just as occurs in the heart and other organs. What results is a decrease in the amount of oxygen available to the brain.

Brain tissue is the most sensitive tissue in the body to oxygen depletion. Brain cells can last only eight minutes without oxygen. The term for damage that occurs due to loss of oxygen is ischemia. Ischemic damage leads to shrinking or the destruction of cells in the brain, and the entire brain begins to lose mass. Atrophy, which occurs in muscles, can also occur in the brain. The final result is a global loss of function that leads to significant cognitive impairment.

Other less common causes of dementia include Lewy-body dementia, Parkinson's disease, heavy metal poisoning, and infections like mad cow disease. Plenty of information exists on these conditions, and they are beyond the scope of this book.

Cognitive Impairment

One of the most difficult medical problems for patients and families to deal with is that of cognitive impairment. The first function to go is "executive function," the process of planning and carrying out a plan. For example, the first sign of dementia is often a loss of the ability to perform a task that one is used to doing automatically, like driving to a familiar place or preparing an old family recipe. Many times, people can cover these early signs by compensating with reminder notes or other strategies. It is easy to write these problems off as normal aging.

The next stage of cognitive impairment involves the instrumental activities of daily living, described in Chapter 2. People begin to lose the ability to perform everyday tasks like using the telephone, shopping, managing finances, or arranging for transportation. It is at this stage that the process crosses into dementia, defined as cognitive impairment that interferes with the ability to live independently and is not attributable to another cause. This is often the stage at which dementia is diagnosed, but sometimes a person may be able to compensate enough to hide the progressive problems. A kind family member or friend may step up and fill in the gaps by providing transportation, meals, or financial management.

This is admirable, but it sometimes allows the underlying problem to carry on without being addressed.

From here, the progression of dementia follows a varied course. People with true Alzheimer's disease tend to progress slowly and deliberately, gradually losing brain function until they become dependent on others for their activities of daily living (ADLs) such as grooming, bathing, dressing, toileting and even feeding. People with vascular dementia tend to follow a more "step-wise" approach, cruising along at the same level for months, but then experiencing a sudden decline in function like the sudden onset of incontinence. This decline establishes the new baseline and the person continues on at this level of function until the next sudden drop. This process may take months or years.

Early Recognition is Key

The earlier dementia is recognized, the sooner a patient can intervene. The medications that are currently used to slow the progression of dementia work best when started at an early stage. Other cognitive and behavioral interventions can be initiated, and studies have shown that preparing one's family and social support network for the onset of advancing dementia can help slow the progression of the disease itself. The first warning signs of dementia should never be ignored or written off as a "senior moment."

There are tests to measure cognitive function at each level. One of the most useful tests in the early stage of cognitive impairment is the clock draw test. It is performed by drawing a circle on a page. The patient is then asked to draw a clock face. Someone with normal cognitive function will develop a plan and then carry it out, exhibiting normal executive function. The patient will usually draw a '12' at the top of the circle, then a '6' at the bottom, followed by a '9' and a '3' in the appropriate location. He or she will then fill in the remainder of the numbers. Next, the examiner will ask the patient to put hands on the clock to indicate a specific time, something like "1:35". The patient with normal cognition will draw a short hand and a long hand in the correct position.

This test will often uncover impaired cognition even in the person who is seemingly carrying out normal daily function at home. People with abnormal executive function will sometimes start with the '12' at the top of the circle, and then number consecutively around the circle, one through eleven. What often happens is they miscalculate the spacing, resulting in incorrect orientation of the numbers, revealing a failure to make a plan. More severe cognitive impairment will result in numbers being placed at random locations around the circle, or outside the circle altogether. A person may get the numbers correct, but when asked to place the hands on the clock, they direct the hands toward the '1' and the '3' for '1:30', or they draw three hands pointing to the 1, 3, and 5 for '1:35'. Any abnormal result is an indication of cognitive impairment.

If you are concerned that a loved one may have cognitive impairment, the clock draw test is an easy exercise to perform at home. If the test is normal, it is very reassuring that your loved one's brain function is healthy. If not, keep the result, make an appointment with your loved one's doctor, and see the doctor together to discuss the issue. You may also want to keep a log of other incidents of memory loss that may seem isolated but are actually indicative of a pattern. This log will be very helpful to the doctor for making a diagnosis of dementia.

As mentioned in the vignette at the beginning of this chapter, the Mini-Mental Status Exam (MMSE) is another short memory test that can be performed in a doctor's office. It is scored on a scale of thirty, and depending on the patient's educational level, the result can confirm the diagnosis of dementia and further classify it into mild, moderate, or severe. The test and instructions for its administration can be found in Appendix F.

Prevention

Alzheimer's disease has no cure and no known treatment or sure-fire preventive strategy. However, more research is being performed on some behavioral and nutritional strategies that can ward off dementia.

The preventive strategy that has the best results in the research so far is regular exercise. People who perform consistent aerobic exercise tend to contract dementia less often. This is likely due to the relationship between exercise and circulatory health. As described above, the brain tissue depends on quality oxygen flow, and if this flow is compromised due to poor circulation, damage can occur over years that is not evident until dementia sets in and it is too late. Commit to regular aerobic exercise that will result in reaching your target heart rate for a sustained amount of time. Thirty minutes of aerobic exercise 4-5 times per week is a great goal.

Certain nutritional supplements have been shown to improve brain health. For a while, gingko was touted as an Alzheimer's prevention supplement, but recent studies have dulled the enthusiasm for this herb and its brain-supporting power. Omega-3 fatty acids are very important for brain health and can be obtained through fresh fish or with a daily supplement. An ingredient in curry is being examined as beneficial to the brain, and other supplements like huperzine may also be helpful, but long-term studies have yet to be published. Consumers should be careful about supplements advertised as "brain boosters." Many of these products contain caffeine, and while they may make you feel more alert, they have no positive impact on brain health. Others do contain some of the ingredients mentioned above, but as with all herbal products, the Food and Drug Administration does not regulate their content or the claims made on the bottle.

In the brain, as with any organ, if you don't use it, you lose it. Commit to exercising your brain in multiple arenas. Keep it as active as possible. Keep up with your favorite mental activity, whether it is reading, puzzles, or card games with friends. It is also important to stretch your brain by learning new activities. This can be frightening, because learning something new can put you in a potentially embarrassing situation. Overcome this fear and take a class or take up a new hobby. Activities that involve physical activity, like dancing, are especially challenging to the brain and therefore make up some of the best mental exercise. Another strategy is to use your non-dominant side more often. If you are right-handed, eat or brush your teeth with your left hand every so often. This will force your brain to stretch itself and will lead to increased blood flow to areas of the brain that may be more stagnant.

Social interaction is also very important for brain health. People who are socially isolated are at much higher risk for the development of dementia. Family interaction can be a source of social engagement, but it is not always reliable in these days of geographically widespread families. Join a local church or religious organization, a local club oriented around a favorite hobby, or an athletic facility like a country club or the YMCA. Taking a class at a local college or community center is another way to find social connection.

Keep Your Brain Young

Dementia is a devastating illness. Its global effects exemplify the loss of independence that inevitably leads to needing long-term care. Caregivers who attend to someone with dementia burn out quickly, leading to nursing home placement in short order. Once dementia has set in, little can be done to slow its effects. Take time now to commit to the principles outlined in this chapter and reduce your chance of contracting the number one cause of long-term placement in a nursing home.

ACTION STEPS

■ Have your doctor or health professional assess your cognitive function with formal memory tests (appendix F)
■ Add Omega-3 to your diet
■ Make an exercise plan for your brain

CHAPTER EIGHT

SHOW ME THE MONEY

Claire, age 72, moved in with her daughter Sandra five years ago after Joe, her husband, died from stomach cancer. Claire received her social security check every month, and she received monthly benefits from the retirement pension Joe earned after thirty years on the police force. She was enrolled with Medicare, and her doctor's visits and most of her medications were covered after she paid her co-payments.

Claire saw her doctor regularly for her rheumatoid arthritis, a condition that at one time was very debilitating for her, but that was now being controlled with medication. For years, she was on corticosteroids to control the arthritis, but her doctor was able to wean her off the steroid medicine prednisone, and transitioned her to newer medicines that had fewer side effects. Claire developed osteoporosis while taking the prednisone, a known consequence or side effect of corticosteroids, so her doctor had her take a calcium supplement three times daily and a bone-building bisphosphonate medication once per week. She was also on three medications to control her high blood pressure. Recently, Claire noticed some difficulty urinating, and her doctor sent her to a urologic specialist for an evaluation.

Claire was diagnosed with obstructive uropathy, a condition that prevents the bladder from emptying completely. She was told that it was probably a consequence of scar tissue inside her abdomen from an emergency C-section she underwent when Sandra was born. The doctor prescribed a new medicine, but Claire continued to have difficulty and never felt like she was able to fully empty her bladder.

One day, Sandra came home from her full-time job at an advertising agency to find Claire hot to the touch and very confused. She rushed her to the ER, where she was diagnosed with a bladder infection and admitted to the hospital. Further testing showed pyelonephritis, a phenomenon that occurs when a urinary tract infection progresses upwards and enters the kidneys. Claire also had acute kidney failure, so intravenous fluids were started.

After several days in the hospital, multiple tests, and consultations with a variety of specialists, it was determined that the infected kidney was simply not working. The urologist decided to place a nephrostomy tube, a catheter that is inserted directly into the kidney and drains out of the back into a collection bag. The doctors also recommended a two week course of IV antibiotics to ensure that the infection was completely cleared.

The hospital social worker explained that Claire's Medicare coverage would not pay for a two week stay in the hospital to complete the antibiotics, but that Medicare would pay for admission to a skilled nursing facility (SNF) for care related to the IV medications. Claire was transferred to a nursing home, where she received the antibiotics through her IV. She also was started on a regimen of physical therapy in anticipation of returning home.

After ten days, Sandra met with Tom, the social services director at the nursing home. He asked Sandra if she had everything ready to take her mother home at the end of the week. "I don't know," she replied. "What do I do about that tube? And she doesn't seem strong enough yet." Tom explained that the Medicare SNF benefit only lasted as long as the patient had a "skilled" need, which was the IV antibiotic in Claire's case.

"Once she finishes those antibiotics, you will need to either take her home or convert to private pay," he said.

"But I thought that Medicare would pay for 100 days in a nursing home after a hospitalization," Sandra protested.

"The benefit can last up to 100 days if necessary, but only if the need for skilled care lasts that long," said Tom. "Since your mother's doctor only recommended two weeks of IV medications, her skilled need ends as soon as her course of antibiotics ends, according to Medicare. I know it's frustrating, but that's just how things work." His matter-of-fact explanation was not encouraging.

"What about the nephrostomy tube? Does that give her a 'skilled need'?" Sandra asked, trying to use terms from this new language that she was struggling to learn along the way.

"Unfortunately, no. There are a limited number of skilled needs that qualify for SNF care under Medicare. Physical therapy, IV medications, treatment of severe skin wounds, and the need for a ventilator machine are a few of them."

"She's getting physical therapy. Doesn't that count?"

"Yes, but only until she meets her goals. The therapist this morning told me that he thought she would reach a plateau in her progress by the end of the week, and once she stops benefiting from daily physical therapy, she no longer qualifies for skilled PT."

Sandra's head was spinning. "How am I supposed to take care of her at home, with her weakness and this tube in her back? I have a full-time job. Won't her health insurance pay for her to stay here longer?"

Tom sighed and replied, "No health insurance plan will pay for room and board in a nursing home once the SNF stay is over. Does she receive a social security check?"

"Yes, it's about $600 per month, and she receives another $1100 per month from her late husband's retirement pension," Sandra said hopefully.

"Well, that will cover about a quarter of her monthly cost. The rest you would have to come up with, unless she has long-term care insurance."

"Long-term care insurance? What is that?"

"If you don't know what it is, then she probably doesn't have it. So I need to know by Friday if you plan to take her home. You could always hire an in-home caregiver and purchase some medical equipment for the home, like a hospital bed, rolling walker, and bedside commode. You'll probably have to cover those costs out-of-pocket as well. Most health insurance plans, even Medicare, just aren't set up to pay for these things."

Financing Your Long Term Care

Many of us are saving for retirement. We work for decades with the dream of amassing enough resources to be able to walk away from a job and do what we want. It is another way we pursue our independence. Yet, money alone cannot guarantee the ability to control our destiny in our later years.

Many people are under the impression that their retirement fund or health insurance will be enough to help them choose where they will live out their final days; often times, they are tragically mistaken.

How Much, and For What?

Before we explore if you will have enough resources to finance your future needs, let us first explore what you will actually have to pay for, which will depend on your level of need. In order to prepare for a variety of potential scenarios, it is crucial to understand the different levels of care and how they are typically financed. The levels of care in the medical system are typically broken down into the following categories, from highest to lowest level of need: inpatient hospitalization, inpatient rehabilitation, skilled nursing facility, long-term, intermediate or custodial care facility (nursing home), assisted living or supportive living, independent living or senior care facility, and living at home.

Inpatient Hospitalization and Inpatient Rehabilitation

When you have a diagnosis that requires hospitalization, Medicare part A (the portion of Medicare into which all U.S. citizens over 65 are required to enroll) and all private medical insurance plans will pay for your stay. The amount for which you will be responsible varies according to each plan, but most of the costs will be covered. As long as the physician documents your need for ongoing hospitalization, the costs will be approved

Hospitals, in an attempt to cut costs, are encouraging doctors to approve shorter and shorter hospital stays. This is partly due to something called the DRG, or Diagnosis-Related Group. The DRG is a system that Medicare created to classify hospital cases into one of about 500 groups that are expected to have similar outcomes. Medicare then pays the hospital a set amount for the patient's hospitalization based on the admitting diagnosis. If the hospital can manage your hospital stay within that amount of money, the hospital earns a profit. If your hospitalization costs the hospital more than the amount they received from the DRG payment, the hospital loses money. This is a simplified explanation, but it highlights why hospitals are motivated to discharge patients quickly, as many of the costs of hospitalization are related to non-medical services like staffing, meals, and housekeeping. The hospital that shaves even one day off of its average length of stay could see an annual benefit in the millions of dollars.

Getting patients out of the hospital can be a very good thing. Hospitals have their own set of risks. Exposure to drug-resistant infections like methicillin-resistant staph aureus (MRSA) is common. Poor sleep due to frequent interruptions for vital signs and medications can take a toll on a patient's health. Limitations on mobility like IV lines, heart monitors, and foley catheters force patients to stay in bed, where they quickly lose their muscle strength, further jeopardizing or delaying their physical rehabilitation. For these reasons, as soon as the acute issue that prompted the hospitalization has been resolved, patients should be discharged.

There is another level of care that takes place in the hospital called inpatient rehabilitation. Any health plan that covers hospitalization will also cover this level of care, usually with the same level of financial responsibility assigned to the patient as with general inpatient hospitalization. Patients who qualify for inpatient rehab must be able to participate in three hours per day of physical, occupational, and speech therapy, six days per week. These patients have usually suffered a spinal cord injury or head injury. They tend to be younger and have excellent rehabilitation potential. Inpatient rehabilitation services are typically overseen by a physician who is board certified in Physical Medicine and Rehabilitation ("PM&R"). This type of service is usually offered only at academic research hospitals, larger community hospitals, or specialized rehabilitation centers in larger cities. You will not find this level of care at a standard nursing home.

Skilled Nursing Facility (SNF)

Most nursing homes survive financially by offering skilled nursing facility (SNF) care. Medicare and most private insurance plans offer a SNF benefit for patients who have undergone a recent hospitalization and are ready to be discharged, but their needs require more attention than they can receive at home. Under Medicare, a patient qualifies for SNF care if he or she has a specific "skilled need". SNF care provides coverage for a stay in a nursing home, including room and board, medications, physical therapy, occupational therapy, speech therapy, wound care, and general nursing care.

What many people do not understand about SNF care is that this is a limited benefit. It only lasts as long as the specific skilled need exists. For example, if you break your hip and undergo a surgical repair, you will likely need two to three weeks of physical and occupational therapy in order to regain your leg strength and return to your previous level of ambulation. As long as you are showing progress with your physical therapy program, Medicare or your health insurance will continue to pay the nursing home at a SNF level; you will not be responsible for your room and board. Once you reach your therapy goals of walking independently, however, you no longer have a "skilled need," so your SNF benefit for the rehabilitation of your hip will terminate. Medicare places a 100 day limit on this benefit, but in most cases, the skilled need is met or resolved long before 100 days.

In some cases, the SNF stay does not have to follow the hospitalization directly. You may not be able to bear weight immediately after a hip surgery and, therefore, unable to participate in a physical therapy rehabilitation program right away. In that case, you could be discharged home until your orthopedic surgeon approved weight bearing exercise, at which time you could return to a SNF facility for a rehabilitation program, and Medicare would cover your stay at the SNF until you met your goals. Admission to the SNF must take place within thirty days of the qualifying hospitalization.

Once the skilled need is met or resolved, most people are discharged home. If the patient wants to stay for any reason, the nursing home will start charging for room and board. This level of care is known as custodial or long-term care.

Custodial Care

People who move into a nursing home permanently receive what is known as custodial care. This is also referred to as intermediate care (ICF) or nursing home level care, depending on where you live. Nursing home residents with custodial care must pay for their own room and board. The monthly fees also cover nursing care, medication administration (not the medications themselves), and other services like daily activities. Your care will be supervised by a doctor who will visit you in the home approximately once per month. If your community doctor makes nursing home rounds, he or she may continue to oversee your care once you move to a nursing home, but many doctors have given up this practice because it is no longer financially feasible to maintain both a nursing home and office practice. Each nursing home has a medical director and a physician who is ultimately responsible for the medical care in the home. You may be assigned to this nursing home doctor if you do not already have your own physician who will come to the nursing home to see you.

Patients who require custodial care need assistance with one or more activities of daily living (ADL's). They are often incontinent or require help with walking or transferring to a wheelchair. On the other hand, they may be physically able to manage their daily activities, but they have cognitive impairment or dementia and are not safe to be left alone. Custodial care nursing homes have certified nurses' aides (CNA's) or licensed practice nurses (LPN's) who perform most of the daily care. There is always at least one registered nurse (RN) in the building during the daytime, but during the evening shifts, the acting director of nursing (DON) is often an LPN who can contact the RN on-call by phone if necessary.

The average cost for a private room in a nursing home in the United States is $70,000 per year. There is a wide range of quality within the nursing home field. Some nursing homes offer gourmet meals, single rooms with balcony views, regular concerts in the facility as well as outings to cultural events, and state-of-the-art entertainment centers in their sitting rooms. These homes tend to have one to two year waiting lists, are very expensive, and are in the minority. Most homes offer adequate, nutritional meals that just meet industry standards, rooms with beds for two to three residents, and activities that mostly take place within the facility with occasional outings to local events.

Paying for nursing home level care can be accomplished several ways. The first way is to pay for everything out of pocket, but for many families, this is simply not an option. Nursing homes will also accept payment from the resident's Social Security benefit, but this usually only covers a portion of the cost. Other retirement payments like monthly pensions can be redirected to the nursing home. Many families also choose to use money put away for retirement, like a 401(k) account, to pay for services.

There is one type of health insurance that will cover the cost of nursing home care, and that is Medicaid. Every state has a Medicaid program, but in order to qualify, your income must fall below a percentage of the poverty line, usually around 150%. For many seniors who are living on a Social Security check alone, it would seem that qualification for this program would be easy. However, Medicaid also takes other assets into account, such as savings accounts, retirement accounts, and your home. If you attempt to give away your assets in order to qualify, you must plan ahead well in advance because most Medicaid programs will take into account any gifts given away in the past five years and still consider those part of your assets.

If you move to a nursing home and your spouse still resides at your current home, Medicaid cannot count your home as one of your assets; otherwise, if you move into a nursing home anticipating that Medicaid will cover your costs, you will have to begin the process of selling your home. This applies even if other family members like your adult children live in that home. Only your spouse can protect your home from being considered in a Medicaid application.

I do not recommend utilizing Medicaid as a means for subsidizing your nursing home costs, if it can be helped. Not all facilities accept Medicaid, and the ones that do tend to provide lower quality of care than the average nursing home. I admire the efforts of facilities that accept Medicaid, but they are faced with the challenges that come with generally poor Medicaid reimbursement for their services. Some are able to offset this lack of funds by admitting residents who pay privately, but often the trend is toward a reduction in the quality of services due to the simple fact that funds are not available. Not only does Medicaid tend to reimburse at a low rate, but they also can delay their payments to nursing homes for six months or more due to bureaucratic red tape.

If you are going to utilize Medicaid as your source of payment, you do not always have to qualify prior to admission to a nursing home. Some nursing homes accept "public aid pending" (PAP) and will help you with your Medicaid application while you live there. Again, these facilities tend to have fewer resources at their disposal and, therefore, the quality of care tends to suffer.

Assisted Living

Assisted Living facilities (ALF) require their residents to have independence with their ADL's in most cases. They cannot have dementia or cognitive impairment. People who live in ALF's need assistance with the IADL's, outlined in chapter 2. The primary services provided by ALF's are meal preparation and help with medications. In many cases, they also provide transportation to doctor's visits, shopping trips, and many in-house amenities like salons, laundry service, and exercise facilities. Most ALF's have single rooms that are equipped with emergency notification alarms and safety equipment like walk-in showers with grab bars. In many ways, living in an assisted living facility is like living in a hotel with some extra services.

ALF's do not require an RN to be present. Most of the staff members have minimal medical training. For this reason, the cost of assisted living is less than the cost of nursing home care. The average cost of an ALF in the U.S. is $ 36,000 per year. As with custodial care nursing homes, there are no medical insurance plans that will cover the cost of a stay in an assisted living facility.

There is one exception, however. In some states, Medicaid will cover the cost of assisted living in a special facility known as a supportive living facility (SLF). In most cases, SLF buildings are of outstanding quality. Supportive living may be an excellent option for those who are already enrolled with Medicaid in their state.

Independent Living

Independent living, sometimes referred to as senior living, is the equivalent of a condominium or apartment specifically designed for older adults. An independent living facility may have added safety features in the units and a central gathering place offering activities geared toward seniors. Exercise or recreational facilities may be present on the premises, and they may also provide a meal plan, although that is not a requirement of the facility. People who live in senior living facilities are independent with their IADL's. They are able, for example, to still manage their own medications and dress and feed themselves without difficulty. They may not be able to drive, but they can arrange for their own transportation. They may not be able to independently manage their finances, but they can delegate the task to a trusted individual and still be part of the decision making process.

Combined Facilities

Some complexes will offer multiple levels of care. In some cases, residents can purchase – without a large increase in cost – an independent living unit with an agreement where they can utilize the assisted living or nursing home level of care as they become more dependent. This arrangement may be a good option for those who have sold their home and know they will likely need care in a long-term facility at some point in the near or not-too-distant future.

In-home Care

For most people, being able to stay in their own home as they age is the ideal situation. That is the point of this entire book. For many, a loss of independence leads to the need for in-home caregivers. Some families are able to rally together and provide the care themselves, but most discover that this can be extremely taxing. A person who is dependent for even one ADL – transferring in and out of bed to a chair, for example – can often employ three people full-time in eight hour shifts, not to mention weekends and holidays. Therefore, for one family member to attempt to take on the needs of a person who is dependent in their ADL function is usually impossible. This has nothing to do with how much the family member cares for his or her loved one. It simply becomes humanly impossible for one person to completely meet the needs of another when he or she is also trying to juggle the requirements of a job and the demands of his or her own immediate family.

Again, medical insurance does not cover the cost of in-home care. It may cover the cost of a visiting nurse for a limited period of time and for a specific need, such as monitoring of blood thinner medication, diabetes care instruction, or wound care, but these visits are likely to occur only two to ten times per month. Health insurance may also cover the cost of a physician's home visit, but only about once per month. Even Medicaid will not cover the cost of an in-home caregiver in most states. This seems counterintuitive, as Medicaid will cover room and board in a nursing home, a cost that is far more expensive than in-home care.

Local departments on aging or senior services may provide meals through a meals-on-wheels program. They may also supply in-home housekeepers for a limited number of hours per week. These assistants have no medical training and cannot offer personal care like bathing, dressing, or even assistance with transfer, because the state agency or department for senior services is not willing to assume liability should anything go wrong. To provide personal care, families must hire an in-home caregiver. These caregivers have a range of certifications. "Non-medical" caregivers will offer personal care like grooming, dressing, bathing, meals, and assistance with transfer and ambulation. They are not, however, qualified to manage medications or other medical care.

How to Pay?

The only insurance that will pay for in-home care, assisted living, or long-term care in a nursing home is long-term care insurance (LTCI). LTC insurance is a policy that will allow you to utilize funds at your discretion towards any of these levels of care. The policy typically pays out at a daily rate until the benefit is used up. Most LTCI covers costs when the individual cannot perform two or more ADL's without significant help. The presence of cognitive impairment or dementia is another trigger that would allow you to use your benefit. Depending on the policy, the benefit could last for months or years. The earlier you buy in, the lower your premium and the larger the benefit you are able to build up. There are some key features to look for in a LTC insurance policy.

Important Features of a Long Term Care Insurance Policy

Portability

LTCI policies vary widely in their cost and benefits offered. Some will cover care in a nursing home or other facility, while others will only cover care at home. More comprehensive policies will allow you to use your benefit in a variety of settings. The first feature to look for in a policy is portability between levels of care. Portability of policy allows you to continue receiving coverage from your long term care insurance even when the circumstances of your care change. For example, if you are in a nursing home and you become well enough to return home, the policy can still cover the necessary equipment or care you may require at home. Indeed, this feature may play a key role in allowing you to make the transition home should you ever need short-term admission to a nursing home.

Elimination Period

LTCI policies usually contain something called the elimination period – the period of time that begins when help is needed and when the insurance company starts paying. It functions like a deductible, but instead of meeting a specified dollar amount before the policy kicks in, you would be required to pay for a certain number of days yourself before receiving compensation through your long term care insurance. The shorter the elimination period, the more expensive the policy. Make sure to clarify the details of the elimination period before making your purchase. In some cases, paying for one day of care per week gives you credit for the entire week, and the shrewd consumer can economically shave seven days off of the elimination period with minimal cost. Some policyholders arrange for free care through family members or other support systems at the beginning of their illness, and since they are not paying for any in-home care, they are unwittingly delaying the start of their policy benefit.

Reasonable and Customary Language

Some policies contain clauses that require the beneficiaries to receive benefits only equal to that which is "reasonable and customary" (R&C). R&C language could limit your benefit in a way that would be unsatisfactory to you. For example, you may have your eye on the fancy nursing home across the street from the forest preserve, but your policy's R&C language only covers the cost of the average nursing homes in town. It is likely that you purchased your LTCI policy so you would have the option of choosing a nicer nursing home, so try to avoid R&C language if you can.

Inflation Protection

Most policies will offer you the option of inserting inflation protection. The younger and healthier you are when you buy your policy, the more important this feature becomes. Inflation protection will increase the amount of your benefit to match or keep up with inflation. Your policy may initially offer a benefit of $300 per day, a reasonable amount for 2010. Fifteen years from now, however, the cost of daily care may increase to $650 per day. If you don't have inflation protection, you will have to come up with the remaining $350/day by yourself once the benefit is utilized. Conventional wisdom states that this feature is especially crucial for anyone purchasing a policy under the age of seventy.

Inflation riders are offered with simple or compound interest. If you can afford it, take the compound interest option as this will increase your benefit at a higher rate. If you are older or expect to utilize your benefit sooner, simple interest may be a better option because it costs less. Inflation protection is sometimes offered with "options" or "future purchase options." This means that you can purchase inflation protection later in the policy. This strategy will result in gradually increasing premiums and should generally be avoided.

One more aspect of inflation protection is the cap. Many policies will cap the inflation protection once the benefit meets a certain level. For example, a policy that offers a $200/day benefit may cap once the benefit doubles to $400/day. Policies without caps are, of course, more expensive, but it is better to have a policy without a cap if possible.

Per Diem vs. Reimbursement

Most LTCI policies offer reimbursement. For example, you pay for your own nursing home or in-home care up front, and at the end of the month, you submit your expenses to the insurance company. A few weeks later, you then receive a check for your qualified expenses. Per diem policies offer a daily reimbursement, paid up front, whether you use the money for health care expenses or not. These policies are naturally more expensive, but they can really pay off if you are relying on unlicensed or unpaid help that would not be considered reimbursable under a reimbursement-based policy. In other words, if you select a reimbursement policy, you will pay a lower premium, but you run the risk of the company rejecting some of your expenses, and you may not be fully reimbursed. If you select a per diem policy, you will pay a higher premium, but you will have more freedom to spend the money as you see fit.

Daily, Weekly, and Monthly Calculation Periods

Policy benefits are calculated based on daily, weekly, or monthly rates. The longer the calculated period, the more flexibility you have. For example, if your policy is for a daily benefit of $200/day, and you only spend $150 on a given day, the $50 is unused and cannot be reimbursed until a new benefit period. Later that week, you may spend $250 in a day, but you will only be reimbursed for $200. On the other hand, if reimbursement is calculated weekly, you would be able to collect the full $400 for the money you spent that week. If you have a monthly policy with a limit of $6000, you can spend $600 on ten separate days during the month, and zero on other days, and you will still receive the full $6000.

Compare and Contrast

Purchasing a LTCI policy is a complex decision and is a form of gambling on the future. Do not rely on the promotional materials for the various policies to guide your decision. Obtain a copy of the actual policy from your agent and get a second opinion. Pay someone if you need to, but have at least two agents or people informed about LTCI look over your policy options and give you advice.

Go with Reputation

Finally, purchase your policy through a reputable company. If the corporation that manages your policy goes bankrupt, you could lose the benefits for which you paid months or years of premiums. Do your best to choose a company that is likely to remain solvent over the next several decades. Consumer

Reports is probably the best place to start when researching the quality of the insurance company and policy.

ACTION STEPS

- Schedule an appointment with your financial advisor, if you have one, to specifically discuss long-term care planning
- Purchase a Long Term Care Insurance plan that fits your needs

CHAPTER NINE

GET BY WITH A LITTLE HELP FROM YOUR FRIENDS

E d, age seventy-five, lived alone in his single-family home. Ed was divorced with three sons, all of whom lived out of state. He saw his doctor only sporadically for medication refills for his enlarged prostate and elevated blood pressure. His younger neighbors next door, Jack and Mary, would check in on him occasionally. Ed took the bus to the grocery store every week for his usual staples that included a six pack of his favorite beer.

One day, Jack was coming home from work when he noticed Ed's mail had been mistakenly delivered to his address instead of to Ed. Ed grabbed the letters and as he slammed the door behind him, yelled "You trying to steal from me?!" Later that week, Mary looked out the window and saw Ed pacing back and forth in his driveway. She went out and found him muttering to himself about "trying to get back to California." She escorted Ed back to his front door and helped him inside. She was shocked by what she saw.

Ed's floor was littered with trash. The refrigerator was open, the spoiled food inside could be smelled from across the room. The bathroom looked like it had not been cleaned in weeks. Mary called Jack, and Jack phoned a friend at the police station. Soon, an ambulance arrived to take Ed to the local emergency room.

Jack and Mary came to the hospital later that evening and found the doctor caring for Ed. "Are you his children?" the doctor asked.

"No, we're just neighbors," Jack replied. "We've never met any of his family."

"Do you know anything about his medical history?" the doctor asked.

"No, we don't," Mary replied, and went on to describe what she found in Ed's home. The doctor explained that Ed would be admitted for observation and treatment for a urinary tract infection that was found on the initial tests.

After several days, Ed had not returned home. Jack phoned the hospital and learned that Ed was transferred to a local nursing home. That weekend, he and Mary went to visit him. When they checked in at the front desk, the administrator called them into her office and began asking what they knew about Ed. He had arrived at the nursing home in a confused state, with the diagnosis of new onset dementia with agitation. The nursing home had been unable to contact any of Ed's family members. Jack and Mary admitted they did not know much about Ed's background, only that he kept to himself most of the time. When Mary described the state of Ed's home on the day he went to the hospital, the administrator gave a knowing nod.

"The Department of Health has been to his house and deemed it uninhabitable for at least two months. It was infested with cockroaches and they're having it fumigated next week. Ed won't be able to return there."

"What's going to happen?" asked Jack.

"Well, Ed has been diagnosed with dementia and is not really able to make decisions for himself. We need someone to act as his guardian." She leaned forward and eyed each of them.

Jack glanced at Mary. "I don't think we could take on that responsibility," he said. "We only know him as neighbors; we don't know anything really personal about him."

"Then unless we can reach some family," the administrator replied, "we're going to have to apply for state guardianship."

Be Realistic

Many people expect that when they become ill, their family will have the resources to step up and fill in the gaps. Often, this is the case at the beginning of an illness. Family members rise to the occasion willingly, preparing meals, going grocery shopping, taking shifts in the home, and accompanying their family member to doctor's visits. This works for a while, but when the needs become extended, family members need to get back to their daily life.

If you lose your independence in one ADL, you may be able to get by with partial assistance from a family member who lives with you or visits daily. Once you lose the ability to perform two or more ADL's independently, you will likely need 24 hour care. A family member who singlehandedly attempts to care for a loved one with this level of need is in for a rude awakening. Often the needs like assistance to the bathroom extend into the night. This arrangement is especially difficult in the setting of dementia, where agitation and wandering can last all night long, and no one gets any sleep. It is possible to employ three people full-time working eight hour shifts, just to care for one person with two or more ADL needs. When one person tries to take this on, it rarely works. This has nothing to do with how much the caregiver loves their family member. It is just humanly impossible for one person to perform a job of that magnitude.

Keep in mind that we reap what we sow Dan Buettner, author of *The Blue Zones: Lessons for Living Longer from Those Who've Lived the Longest* observes that, in cultures where people live well into their 100's, families tend to care for each other and maintain good relations. Nursing homes only exist for those with extreme disability. Aging is seen as a part of life, and families model the practice of caring for their parents. He says, "I am doing my best to care for my aging parents, not only because it is the right thing to do, but because I am setting an example for what I hope my children will do for me someday."

Prepare your caregivers

If you want to rely on family or friends to care for you should you develop the need for help, start to talk about it well in advance. Find out who might be willing, in the event of a crisis, to move in with you for a while. If the answer is no one, broach the subject of moving in with them. If you discuss these options prior to a crisis, the chances of making it happen increase dramatically. Last minute living arrangements tend to lead to confusion and bitterness.

Find Your Advocate

Perhaps the most important step to take in establishing your social support structure is identifying your health advocate. A health advocate is someone you trust to travel with you in your health care journey. He or she can help you think ahead about items, services, or adjustments you may need for the future. They can ask the questions you don't ask because of fear or forgetfulness. Your health advocate may be able to recognize changes in your health status before you recognize them yourself. Having a reliable health advocate increases your chances of heading off a crisis before it happens.

The most important role your health advocate can play is that of Durable Power of Attorney for Health Care (DPAHC), also referred to as an advance directive or "health care power of attorney." Your DPAHC should be someone you trust to make health care decisions for you if you were ever in a situation where you could not express your wishes (for example, a car accident or severe stroke has left your father unable to speak or communicate in any way). Establishing your DPAHC is a simple process.

First, decide on who you believe would be the best person to handle such a responsibility. The DPAHC needs to be just one person, but successor agents can be chosen should the first designated person be unable to complete his or her duties. Next, ask that person if he or she would be willing to act as your DPAHC. If the person agrees, locate the DPAHC form for your state – the website for your state's attorney general will most likely have the DPAHC form that you can download at no cost, along with instructions on how to correctly complete the form (for example, you may be required to have witnesses to your signature). In most states, you can complete the DPAHC without assistance from a lawyer or doctor. If you do seek an attorney's help on this matter, it would not be uncommon for you to take care of the DPAHC issue along with other estate planning matters, such as creating your last will and testament, creating a revocable trust, etc. Your DPAHC may not need to sign it, but it is recommended.

Once the forms are complete, make several copies. Give one to your DPAHC, one to your primary doctor, one to your lawyer (if applicable), one copy each to your successor agents (if applicable), and keep two copies for yourself. **The next step is perhaps the most important. Have a conversation with your DPAHC about your wishes.** This is probably best accomplished by starting with what you value most when it comes to your health care. Once your values have been established, this will guide your conversation about specific interventions you may or may not want.

It is not necessary to cover every possible scenario in the discussions you have with your DPAHC. If the person you've chosen has a good understanding on what you value, he or she will probably make the right decisions on your behalf. If you want help with this conversation, schedule an appointment with your doctor that you and your DPAHC can attend together. Ask for extra time when you make the appointment and let your doctor know that you want to discuss DPAHC matters as opposed to coming in for follow-up appointment regarding a health issue. Some areas of the country have "advance care planning" facilitators who can also help with this process. LaCrosse, Wisconsin is one example, where a citywide effort called "Respecting Choices" led to completion of advance care planning documents for over 90% of the city's residents.

What If I Don't Have Anyone?

There are those in a situation where they have no family or friend they believe would be willing to play the role of health care advocate. If you are in that situation, and you were to have a health crisis from which you did not recover, and you were unable to voice your wishes, then decisions about your health care would likely fall to your state's Office of Guardianship. Applying for guardianship is a lengthy process and is not to your advantage. There is no guarantee that that guardian assigned to your care would know anything about you or make decisions that are in line with your wishes. You want to avoid this scenario.

If you are like Ed, in the above scenario, and you do not have anyone you can trust as a health advocate, your risk for a health crisis in the near future is very high. Social isolation is linked to many types of health problems and to a high rate of mortality among older adults. Do what you can to develop new, trusting relationships, even if past relationships have been severely damaged. Join a church, synagogue, or other religious community. Join a social club or local community center. Most cities and towns have a Department on Aging or

Senior Services Department that can point you in the right direction.

Private organizations also exist that provide "health advocacy" for a fee. These companies may define themselves as "Health Care Advocates," or they may provide services called "care management" or "geriatric case management." These services are private pay and not covered by insurance, but if you have no one else to act in this important role on your behalf, this may be a good option for you.

Legal vs. Medical

Keep in mind that the DPAHC is not the same thing as a power of attorney for property. You will also need to select someone you trust to manage your financial and estate affairs if you are unable to express your wishes and desires regarding your finances and assets. This could be the same person as your DPAHC, but many people choose two different people due to fears about creating a conflict of interest or imposing an undue burden on the individual who has been asked to make both financial and health care decisions. I'll never forget my patient who chose his current wife as the power of attorney for his estate, and his ex-wife as his power of attorney for health care. "This way, neither one can kill me to get my money," he reasoned.

Talk

The most important thing you can do to prepare your social support system for future needs is to talk. Talk about it! This is always a difficult conversation to have – nobody wants to have a serious conversation about getting old, possibly losing your ability to engage in one or more ADLs, and not being able to speak should a sudden health crisis or tragedy strike. But you must let your loved ones know how you would want to be cared for should that happen. Share what you are afraid of. This may include feeling like a burden to them or creating resentment in them as they adjust their lives to care for you. Talk about what is most important to you. Describe your ideal situation, or what you absolutely refuse to let happen. This conversation is not a one-time event. It is an ongoing process that constitutes many conversations which may also change as your health status changes. Issues that you were adamant about avoiding at one stage may now seem natural and reasonable at the next stage, or vice versa.

ACTION STEPS

- Choose your Health Advocate
- Complete Durable Power of Attorney for Health Care (DPAHC) and give copies to appropriate recipients (appendix H)
- Have a conversation with your Health Advocate about your health care wishes

CONCLUSION

Nursing homes serve an important role in the lives of many older adults, but you can choose not to fall into the nursing home trap. Physical, social, and financial threats to independence will increase as you age, but you can take steps today to ensure that these threats do not push you into the spiral of dependent living. I have attempted to identify the key causes of nursing home placement so that you may develop strategies for avoiding them. Recognizing that a major lifestyle overhaul is unrealistic and unnecessary, I offer steps that do not require extraordinary efforts, but that focus on the most important aspects of independent living.

No matter your stage of life, this book can help you prepare for the future. Choose the steps in this book that make sense to you and carry them out. Maintaining your independence is best accomplished by developing small habits that will preserve the functions that are at greatest risk from the effects of aging. I hope that I have offered you some practical strategies that will enable you to efficiently and effectively incorporate these habits into your lifestyle. We cannot control the fact that we are getting older, but we can control the path we take as we age. Make the choice today to walk the road well traveled.

A NOTE
FROM THE AUTHOR

As a physician, I have dedicated my life to studying the human body. Everything I learn convinces me that we were created by God. The miraculously intricate design of our body is proof enough for me. The focus of this book is to help you maximize your care for your body, but I am convinced that our health is more than physical. We were clearly created for relationship, and physical health without emotional and spiritual health results only in depression and despair.

If we achieve emotional and spiritual health through relationships, why do they also cause pain? We are imperfect beings. Trusting in a flawed, fellow human to rectify our spiritual and emotional shortages always ends in disappointment. So are we without hope? Thankfully, no. There is hope for complete fulfillment. God, our creator, desires relationship with us. I know God is relational because we are, and how could a non-relational being create relational beings?

Fulfillment and joy is found in relationship with God. Explore this. Talk to God. In my experience, He listens and responds. I have learned the most about God through the teachings of Jesus. Not necessarily Christianity, or Christian culture, but the person of Jesus as described in the Gospel Letters of the New Testament. As you read the short letters by Matthew, Mark, Luke and John, you will find that Jesus' perspective on life and health is unique in history. More importantly, Jesus made the bold claim that he is the way to God and the path to true life.

It may be well with your physical body, but is it well with your soul? If you cannot answer with a firm 'yes,' investigate Jesus' claim as the source of true fulfillment. I did not make that claim, he did. Perhaps the most important question you can answer in life is whether Jesus' claim is valid. I investigated for myself, and my life was completely changed. I do not include this to sound preachy. Spiritually speaking, I am simply a beggar who found free bread, and if you are spiritually hungry, I want to share it with you.

APPENDIX A

Activities of Daily Living (ADL) Assessment

ADL Questionnaire

1. Can you eat ...

2   without help (able to feed yourself completely);

1   with some help (need help with cutting, etc.); or

0   are you completely unable to feed yourself?

2. Can you dress and undress yourself ...

2   without help (able to pick out clothes, dress and undress yourself);

1   with some help; or

0   are you completely unable to dress and undress yourself?

3. *Can you take care of your own appearance, for example, combing your hair and (for men) shaving ...*

2   without help;

1   with some help; or

0   are you completely unable to maintain your appearance yourself?

4. *Can you walk or transport yourself ...*

2   without help (except from a cane);

1   with some help from a person or with the use of a walker, crutches, or wheelchair etc; or

0   are you completely unable to walk?

5. *Can you get in and out of bed ...*

2   without any help or aids;

1   with some help (either from a person or with the aid of some device); or

0   are you totally dependent on someone else to lift you?

6. *Can you take a bath or shower ...*

2   without help;

1   with some help (need help getting in and out of the tub, or need special attachments on the tub); or

0   are you completely unable to bathe yourself?

7. *Do you ever have trouble getting to the bathroom on time?*

2   No

0   Yes

1   Have a catheter or colostomy

8. If yes, how often do you wet or soil yourself (either day or night)?

1   Once or twice a week

0   Three times a week or more

Instrumental ADL Questionnaire

1. Can you use the telephone ...

2   without help, including looking up numbers and dialing;

1   with some help (can answer phone or dial operator in an emergency, but need a special phone or help in getting the number or dialing); or

0   are you completely unable to use the telephone?

2. Can you get to places out of walking distance ...

2   without help (drive your own car, or travel alone on buses, or taxis);

1   with some help (need someone to help you or go with you when traveling); or

0   are you unable to travel unless emergency arrangements are made for a specialized vehicle like an ambulance?

3. Can you go shopping for groceries or clothes...

2   without help (taking care of all shopping needs yourself, assuming you had transportation);

1   with some help (need someone to go with you on all shopping trips); or

0   are you completely unable to do any shopping?

4. Can you prepare your own meals ...

2   without help (plan and cook full meals yourself);

1   with some help (can prepare some things but unable to cook full meals yourself); or

0   are you completely unable to prepare any meals?

5. Can you do your housework ...

2   without help (can clean floors, etc.);

1   with some help (can do light housework but need help with heavy work); or

0   are you completely unable to do any housework?

6. Can you take your own medicine ...

2   without help (in the right doses at the right time);

1   with some help (able to take medicine if someone prepares it for you and/or reminds you to take it); or

0   are you completely unable to take your medicines?

7. Can you handle your own money ...

2   without help (write checks, pay bills, etc.);

1   with some help (manage day-to-day buying but need help with managing your checkbook and paying your bills); or

0   are you completely unable to handle money?

SCORING

ADL Questionnaire

12-14   Low risk of nursing home placement within the next two years

9-11   Moderate risk of nursing home placement within the next two years

5-8   High risk of nursing home placement within the next year

0-4   Likely already reside in nursing home or have 24-hour care at home

IADL Questionnaire

12-14   Low risk of nursing home placement within the next five years

9-11   Low risk of nursing home placement within the next three years

5-8   Moderate risk of nursing home placement within the next three years

0-4   High risk of nursing home placement within the next three years

Source:
Older Americans Resources and Services Program of the
Duke University Center for the Study of Aging and Human
Development; Durham, NC 27710

APPENDIX B

Quadriceps Exercises

1. Quad Extension

Do this every time you sit down.

Sit back in the chair with good posture. Straighten and raise the leg, hold it for a slow count to10, then slowly lower it.

Repeat this 10 times with each leg

If this can be done easily, repeat the exercises with a weight on the ankle (buy ankle weights from a sports shop or improvise, for example with a can of peas in a carrier bag wrapped around the ankle).

2. Leg Lift

With one leg bent at the knee, hold the other leg straight and lift the foot six inches off the bed.

Hold for a slow count of 5 then lower. Repeat with each leg 5 times every morning and evening.

3. Quad Clench

During the day, whether standing or sitting, get into the habit of clenching and releasing the quadriceps muscles. By constantly stimulating the muscles, they become stronger.

Source:
Arthritis Research UK
www.arc.org.uk

APPENDIX C

Urinary Incontinence Risk Assessment

Risk Factors

1. What is your gender?

1   Female
0   Male

2. What is your age?

2   Over 80
1   Over 65
0   Under 65

3. Have you delivered a child vaginally?

2   Yes, over the age of 30
1   Yes, under the age of 30
0   No

4. Have you had a hysterectomy?

1   Yes

0   No

5. Do you smoke?

1   Yes

0   No

6. What is your BMI?

2   Over 28

1   Between 24 and 28

0   24 or under

7. Do you have diabetes?

1   Yes

0   No

8. Have you had 2 or more urinary tract infections in the past year?

1   Yes

0   No

High risk 8-11

Moderate risk 5-7

Low risk 0-4

APPENDIX D

Adequate Intakes for Calcium

Age	Male	Female	Pregnant	Lactating
Birth to 6 months	210 mg	210 mg		
7-12 months	270 mg	270 mg		
1-3 years	500 mg	500 mg		
4-8 years	800 mg	800 mg		
9-13 years	1,300 mg	1,300 mg		
14-18 years	1,300 mg	1,300 mg	1,300 mg	1,300 mg
19-50 years	1,000 mg	1,000 mg	1,000 mg	1,000 mg
50+ years	1,200 mg	1,200 mg		

Source: National Institutes of Health, Office of Dietary Supplements Dietary Supplement Fact Sheet, Calcium

Adequate Intake of Vitamin D

Age	Children	Men	Women	Pregnancy	Lactation
Birth to 13 years	5 mcg (200 IU)				
14-18 years		5 mcg (200 IU)	5 mcg (200 IU)	5 mcg (200 IU)	5 mcg (200 IU)
19-50 years		5 mcg (200 IU)	5 mcg (200 IU)	5 mcg (200 IU)	5 mcg (200 IU)
51-70 years		10 mcg (400 IU)	10 mcg (400 IU)		
71+ years		15 mcg (600 IU)	15 mcg (600 IU)		

These values are in dispute and many clinicians and experts are recommending higher levels of vitamin D. These values could likely be doubled safely. The Food and Nutrition Board will release new recommendations as of May 2010.

Source: National Institutes of Health, Office of Dietary Supplements Dietary Supplement Fact Sheet: Vitamin D

Select Sources of Vitamin D

Food	IUs per serving*
Cod liver oil, 1 tablespoon	1,360
Salmon (sockeye), cooked, 3 ounces	794
Mackerel, cooked, 3 ounces	388
Tuna fish, canned in water, drained, 3 ounces	154
Milk, nonfat, reduced fat, and whole, vitamin D-fortified, 1 cup	115-124
Orange juice fortified with vitamin D, 1 cup (check product labels, as amount of added vitamin D varies)	100
Yogurt, fortified with 20% of the DV for vitamin D, 6 ounces (more heavily fortified yogurts provide more of the DV)	80
Margarine, fortified, 1 tablespoon	60
Sardines, canned in oil, drained, 2 sardines	46
Liver, beef, cooked, 3.5 ounces	46
Ready-to-eat cereal, fortified with 10% of the DV for vitamin D, 0.75-1 cup (more heavily fortified cereals might provide more of the DV)	40

Source: National Institutes of Health, Office of Dietary Supplements

Select Sources of Calcium

Food	Milligrams (mg) per serving	Percent DV*
Yogurt, plain, low fat, 8 ounces	415	42
Sardines, canned in oil, with bones, 3 ounces	324	32
Cheddar cheese, 1.5 ounces	306	31
Milk, nonfat, 8 ounces	302	30
Milk, reduced-fat (2% milk fat), 8 ounces	297	30
Milk, lactose-reduced, 8 ounces**	285-302	29-30
Milk, whole (3.25% milk fat), 8 ounces	291	29
Milk, buttermilk, 8 ounces	285	29
Mozzarella, part skim, 1.5 ounces	275	28
Yogurt, fruit, low fat, 8 ounces	245-384	25-38
Orange juice, calcium-fortified, 6 ounces	200-260	20-26
Tofu, firm, made with calcium sulfate, ½ cup***	204	20
Salmon, pink, canned, solids with bone, 3 ounces	181	18
Pudding, chocolate, instant, made with 2% milk, ½ cup	153	15

Food	Milligrams (mg) per serving	Percent DV*
Cottage cheese, 1% milk fat, 1 cup unpacked	138	14
Tofu, soft, made with calcium sulfate, ½ cup***	138	14
Spinach, cooked, ½ cup	120	12
Ready-to-eat cereal, calcium-fortified, 1 cup	100-1,000	10-100
Instant breakfast drink, various flavors and brands, powder prepared with water, 8 ounces	105-250	10-25
Frozen yogurt, vanilla, soft serve, ½ cup	103	10
Turnip greens, boiled, ½ cup	99	10
Kale, cooked, 1 cup	94	9
Kale, raw, 1 cup	90	9
Ice cream, vanilla, ½ cup	85	8.5
Soy beverage, calcium-fortified, 8 ounces	80-500	8-50
Chinese cabbage, raw, 1 cup	74	7
Tortilla, corn, ready-to-bake/fry, 1 medium	42	4
Tortilla, corn, ready-to-bake/fry, one 6" diameter	37	4

Food	Milligrams (mg) per serving	Percent DV*
Sour cream, reduced fat, cultured, 2 tablespoons	32	3
Bread, white, 1 ounce	31	3
Broccoli, raw, ½ cup	21	2
Bread, whole-wheat, 1 slice	20	2
Cheese, cream, regular, 1 tablespoon	12	1

Source: National Institutes of Health, Office of Dietary Supplements

APPENDIX E

Bone Mineral Density

Recommendations for Testing

Your healthcare provider may recommend a BMD test if you are:

- A postmenopausal woman under age 65 with one or more risk factors for osteoporosis
- A man age 50-70 with one or more risk factors for osteoporosis
- A woman age 65 or older, even without any risk factors
- A man age 70 or older, even without any risk factors
- A woman or man after age 50 who has broken a bone
- A woman going through menopause with certain risk factors
- A postmenopausal woman who has stopped taking estrogen therapy (ET) or hormone therapy (HT)

Some other reasons your healthcare provider may recommend a BMD test:

- Long-term use of certain medications including steroids (for example, prednisone and cortisone), some anti-seizure medications, Depo-Provera® and aromatase inhibitors (for example, anastrozole, brand name Arimidex®)
- A man receiving certain treatments for prostate cancer
- A woman receiving certain treatments for breast cancer
- Overactive thyroid gland (hyperthyroidism) or taking high doses of thyroid hormone medication
- Overactive parathyroid gland (hyperparathyroidism)
- X-ray of the spine showing a fracture or bone loss
- Back pain with a possible fracture
- Significant loss of height
- Loss of sex hormones at an early age, including early menopause
- Having a disease or condition that can cause bone loss (such as rheumatoid arthritis or anorexia nervosa)

APPENDIX F

Cognitive Function Tests

Clock Draw Test (CDT)

1) Inside the circle, draw the hours of a clock as they normally appear
2) Place the hands of the clock to represent the time:"ten minutes after eleven o'clock"

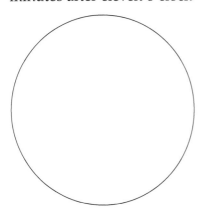

Normal

- No errors in the task
- Mildly impaired spacing of times
- Draws times outside circle
- Turns page while writing so that some numbers appear upside down
- Draws in lines (spokes) to orient spacing

Early Abnormalities

- Minute hand points to 10
- Writes "10 after 11"
- Unable to make any denotation of time
- Moderately poor spacing

Abnormal

- Omits numbers
- Perseveration: repeats circle or continues
- on past 12 to 13, 14, 15, etc.
- Right-left reversal: numbers drawn counterclockwise
- Dysgraphia: unable to write numbers accurately

Severely Abnormal

- No attempt at all
- No semblance of a clock at all
- Writes a word or name

Source: Palmer RM, Meldon SW. Acute Care. In: Principles of Geriatric Medicine and Gerontology, 5th edition, 2003. Eds. Hazzard WR et al. McGraw-Hill Pub. pp 157-168

The Mini-Cog Assessment Instrument for Dementia

This simple test is most accurate when administered by a trained professional like a physician or psychologist. However, it can be used be a layperson to screen for abnormalities in memory and thinking.

Administration

1. Instruct the patient to listen carefully and remember 3 unrelated words. Examples are "ball, flag and tree" or "apple, table and penny." Then ask the patient to repeat the words.
2. Administer the Clock Draw Test (see previous page)
3. Ask the patient to repeat the 3 previously presented words.

Scoring

Give 1 point for each recalled word after the CDT distractor. Score 1–3.

Score = 0 positive screen for dementia

Score =1 or 2 with an abnormal CDT positive screen for dementia

Score =1 or 2 with a normal CDT negative screen for dementia

Score = 3 negative screen for dementia

The CDT is considered normal if all numbers are present in the correct sequence and position, and the hands readably display the requested time.

*This test does not diagnose dementia. It merely screens for those patients who may need further testing to evaluate their cognitive deficits.

Source: Borson S, Scanlan J, Brush M, Vitaliano P, Dokmak A. The mini-cog: a cognitive "vital signs" measure for dementia screening in multi-lingual elderly. Int J Geriatr Psychiatry 2000; 15(11): 1021–1027.

APPENDIX G

Screening Tests for Depression in Older Adults

Many "depression scales" are used by geriatricians to identify patients who may be depressed. Some of the questions are so depressing, however, that the patients who weren't depressed before taking this test may end up depressed afterwards!

A useful (and scientifically valid) method to screen for depression is to ask the simple question:

"Do you often feel sad or depressed?"

A 'yes' answer warrants further investigation with your physician. Make an appointment to specifically talk about this issue.

The following test is the most commonly used depression screening tool, but the diagnosis of depression can only be made by a physician through a multi-question interview in the context of the patient's medical, social and spiritual history.

Geriatric Depression Scale (Short Form)

Choose the best answer for how you felt over the past week.

1. Are you basically satisfied with your life? YES/**NO**
2. Have you dropped many of your activities and interests? **YES**/NO
3. Do you feel that your life is empty? **YES**/NO
4. Do you often get bored? **YES**/NO
5. Are you in good spirits most of the time? YES/**NO**
6. Are you afraid that something bad is going to happen to you? **YES**/NO
7. Do you feel happy most of the time? YES/**NO**
8. Do you often feel helpless? **YES**/NO
9. Do you prefer to stay at home, rather than going out and doing new things? **YES**/NO
10. Do you feel you have more problems with memory than most? **YES**/NO
11. Do you think it is wonderful to be alive now? YES/**NO**
12. Do you feel pretty worthless the way you are now? **YES**/NO
13. Do you feel full of energy? YES/**NO**
14. Do you feel that your situation is hopeless? **YES**/NO
15. Do you think that most people are better off than you are? **YES**/NO

Score 1 point for each bolded answer

A score above 5 suggests depression

Source: Sheikh JI, Yesavage JA. Geriatric Depression Scale: recent evidence and development of a shorter version. Clin Gerontol. 1986; 5:165-172.

APPENDIX H

Resources for Advance Care Planning

Durable Power of Attorney for Health Care (DPAHC)

This, in my opinion, is the most useful of the advance care planning documents.

Each state has a different form. You can usually find your state's form at the website for the State Department of Public Health.

Or, visit the following website for state-specific documents and instructions: *www.nationalhealthcaredecisionsday.org/takeaction/advance_directive*

Living Will

There are many versions of this document, but if you want to complete one, there is a form called "Five Wishes" that meets the legal requirements of most states.

You can find "Five Wishes" at the following website: *www.agingwithdignity.org*

Do Not Resuscitate (DNR)/ Physician Orders for Life-Sustaining Treatment (POLST)

DNR and POLST are orders written by a physician with the patient's consent that will dictate the medical approach in very specific situations. Each state has a different DNR form, and only some states have instituted POLST forms. Search your state's Department of Public Health website if you want to see the form.

You must meet with your physician in order to complete a DNR or POLST form.

Advance Care Planning Counseling

Some hospitals and health care systems offer voluntary counseling sessions with trained professionals who can help you sort through the documentation you will need to ensure that your wishes are met. To find this type of services, a good place to start is Respecting Choices. This organization is a national leader in promoting advance care planning.

www.respectingchoices.org

GLOSSARY OF TERMS

Activities of Daily Living (ADL)

Five basic activities of self-care that impact daily independence and function. They are bathing, dressing, feeding one's self, toileting, and transfer (from bed to standing, chair to wheelchair, etc). Loss of independence with one or more ADL often leads to nursing home placement.

Advance directive

Any document that allows patients to express wishes regarding future health care decisions. These include Durable Power of Attorney for Health Care, Living Will, Do Not Resuscitate orders, and basic Advance Directives.

Alzheimer's disease

A chronic, progressive illness with some hereditary component that usually strikes people over the age of 70. It is the leading cause of dementia in the United States.

Assisted Living Facility (ALF)

A senior living center that provides basic needs such as meals and medication management. Most ALF residents require assistance with some IADLs, but they are independent with their ADLs.

Cerebrovascular disease

A disorder of circulation in the brain that can lead to strokes or vascular dementia. It is often caused by years of high blood pressure or high cholesterol

Cognitive impairment

Loss of memory or thinking function that does not impact daily living. It may develop into Alzheimer's disease or it may be a function of normal aging, or both

Compression fracture

A fracture of one of the vertebrae in which the bone collapses in on itself. Multiple compression fractures lead to kyphosis, or spinal curvature leading to stooped posture

Congestive heart failure (CHF)

A loss of heart function leading to inefficient pumping of blood with each heartbeat. CHF is usually caused by years of damage to the heart muscle from high blood pressure or high cholesterol. Other causes include disorders of the heart valves and heavy alcohol use.

Dementia

A term for loss of cognitive function that impacts daily life. The most common cause of dementia is Alzheimer's disease, but other causes include vascular (circulatory) disease in the brain, Parkinson's disease, and Lewy-body dementia.

Do Not Resuscitate (DNR)

A physician order to refrain from attempts at cardiopulmonary resuscitation (CPR) in the event of cardiac arrest. The DNR only applies when the heart stops beating or the patient stops breathing. Many states have an official DNR form that is transportable across levels of care: hospital, nursing home, ambulance, home, etc.

Durable Power of Attorney for Health Care (DPAHC)

The person you choose to make health care decisions on your behalf if you are incapacitated and unable to express your own wishes

Functional incontinence

A type of incontinence that is caused by multiple factors and is related to immobility. The bladder is functioning normally, but other factors like muscle weakness prevent the patient from traveling to the bathroom on time

Hemorrhagic stroke

A stroke that occurs when a blood vessel ruptures and bleeds into part of the brain

Independent Living Facility (ILF)

A senior living center that provides optional services such as meals and safety surveillance. ILFs do not offer nursing care for chronic medical conditions. ILFs function similarly to a dormitory.

In-Home Care

Caregiving services offered in the home. These services may or may not include personal care or medical care.

Instrumental Activities of Daily Living (IADL)

Eight activities that enable people to live independently. They are managing money, managing medications, preparing meals, grocery shopping, arranging for transportation, using a telephone, performing housework, and doing laundry.

Ischemic stroke

A stroke that occurs when a portion of the brain is starved for oxygen, usually due to a blockage in the brain's circulation from a blood clot or a cholesterol plaque

Living Will

A document that allows patients to indicate specific wishes related to their health care, specifically regarding life-sustaining treatment in the context of permanent incapacity of consciousness

Long-term Care Facility

A general term for senior living facilities, but often refers specifically to nursing home level of care

Long-term care insurance (LTCI)

Insurance that specifically pays for care in a nursing home, assisted living, or in-home medical care. It is a separate policy from health insurance or life insurance.

Medicare Part A

The portion of Medicare that is accessible to all citizens over 65 and those with certain disabilities. Part A covers the expenses related to a hospitalization, which may include a rehabilitation stay in a skilled nursing facility

Medicare Part B

The portion of Medicare that covers outpatient visits and procedures. Part B is optional and usually involves small premiums and copayments.

Medicare Part C

Also known as Medicare Advantage, a program that allows private insurance companies to provide care for Medicare recipients using mostly Medicare funds

Medicare Part D

The portion of Medicare that pays for certain prescription drugs

Nursing Home

A long-term care facility that provides a specific level of medical care. In addition to providing meals and medication management, residents receive care from a registered nurse for chronic conditions. They also receive a higher level of personal assistance from certified nurses aides. Most nursing home residents need assistance with two or more ADLs.

Skilled Nursing Facility (SNF)

Nursing home with a specific number of nurses trained in specific skills. Skilled nursing facilities offer rehabilitation, usually in the form of physical and occupational therapy. Medicare will pay for a limited number of days in a SNF, depending on the patient's specific need.

Occupational Therapy (OT)

A discipline of rehabilitation that emphasizes engagement in meaningful activities of daily life. OT focuses on specific abilities, such as the ability to feed one's self, get in and out of a car, and open a can of food.

Osteopenia

Loss of bone density that is a precursor to osteoporosis. Patients with osteopenia usually engage in basic bone-building activities like weight-bearing exercise and taking calcium.

Osteoporosis

Loss of bone density and structure that dramatically increases the risk for fracture

Overflow incontinence

A type of incontinence caused by loss of sensation in the bladder. Damaged nerves fail to send the signal that the bladder needs to be emptied.

Physical Therapy (PT)

A discipline of rehabilitation that uses specially designed exercises and equipment to help patients regain or improve their physical abilities. PT emphasizes independence with general mobility.

Quadriceps

A group of four muscles in front of the thigh that is instrumental in maintaining the ability to walk and transfer

Speech Therapy (ST)

A discipline of rehabilitation that seeks to restore basic speech skills, but may also include rehabilitation of swallowing function. ST explores both the physical and cognitive causes of speech deficit.

Stress incontinence

A type of incontinence caused by weakness of the external bladder sphincter. When a patient with stress incontinence laughs, coughs, sneezes, or stands up, the bladder often leak

Stroke

Damage to the brain that occurs due to an interruption of blood flow. Symptoms must last more than twenty-four hours.

Transient ischemic attack (TIA)

An interruption in blood flow to the brain which causes symptoms that last less than 24 hours. Sometimes called a "mini-stroke"

Urge incontinence

A type of incontinence caused by bladder spasms. When the bladder muscles contract, the patient feels the immediate urge to urinate but often cannot travel to the bathroom in time

Urinary sphincter

The muscle that allows one to hold urine in the bladder until it is safe to urinate

ABOUT THE AUTHOR

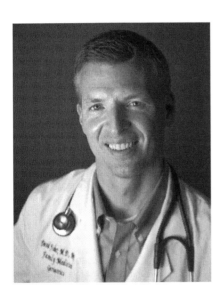

David Fisher, MD, is a family physician and geriatrician. He is a graduate of Rush Medical College in Chicago and completed his geriatrics training at Wake Forest University in North Carolina. Dr. Fisher's passion is to enhance his patient's health by directing them to the most effective practical steps for aging well.

Additional copies can be purchased at www.doctorfisher.com

7449167R0

Made in the USA
Lexington, KY
24 November 2010